My Mediterranean Cooking Guide

Super Tasty and Delicious
Side Dishes Recipes

Ben Cooper

Table of Contents

6

Apples and Pomegranate Salad

Preparation Time: 10 minutes
Cooking Time: 0 minutes
Servings: 4

Ingredients:

3 big apples, cored and cubed
1 cup pomegranate seeds
3 cups baby arugula
1 cup walnuts, chopped
1 tbsp. olive oil
1 tsp. white sesame seeds
2 tbsp. apple cider vinegar
Salt and black pepper to the taste

Directions:

1.In a bowl, mix the apples with the arugula and the rest of the ingredients, toss and serve cold.

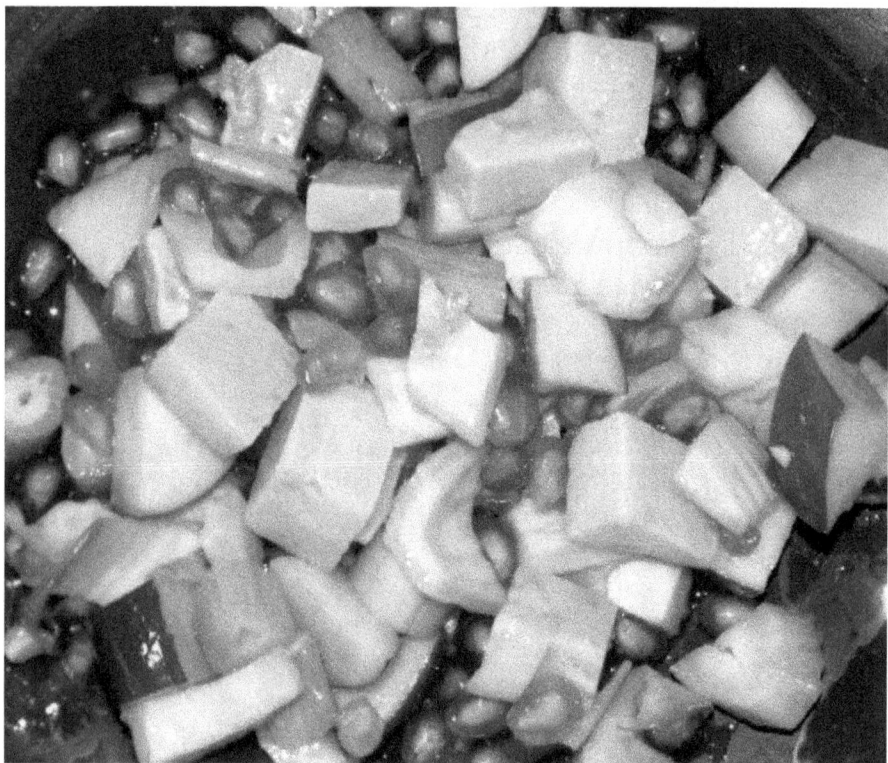

Cranberry Bulgur Mix Preparation

Preparation Time: 10 minutes
Cooking Time: 0 minutes
Servings: 4

Ingredients:

1 and ½ cups hot water
1 cup bulgur
Juice of ½ lemon
4 tbsp. cilantro, chopped
½ cup cranberries, chopped
1 and ½ tsp. curry powder
¼ cup green onions, chopped
½ cup red bell peppers, chopped
½ cup carrots, grated
1 tbsp. olive oil
A pinch of salt and black pepper

Directions:

1.Put bulgur into a bowl, add the water, stir, cover, leave aside for 10 minutes, fluff with a fork and transfer to a bowl.

2.Add the rest of the ingredients, toss, and serve cold.

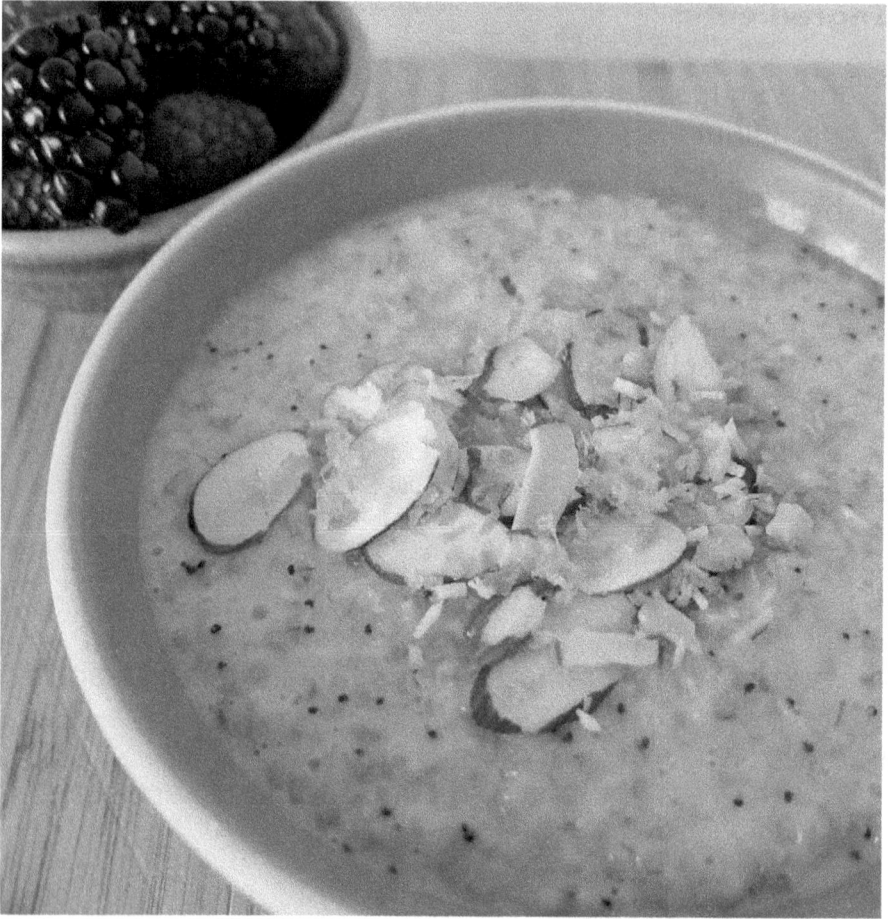

Chickpeas, Corn and Black Beans Salad

Preparation Time: 10 minutes
Cooking Time: 0 minutes
Servings: 4

Ingredients:

1 and ½ cups canned black beans, drained and rinsed
½ tsp. garlic powder
2 tsp. chili powder
A pinch of sea salt and black pepper
1 and ½ cups canned chickpeas, drained and rinsed
1 cup baby spinach
1 avocado, pitted, peeled and chopped
1 cup corn kernels, chopped
2 tbsp. lemon juice
1 tbsp. olive oil
1 tbsp. apple cider vinegar
1 tsp. chives, chopped

Directions:

1.In a salad bowl, combine the black beans with the garlic powder, chili powder and the rest of the ingredients, toss and serve cold.

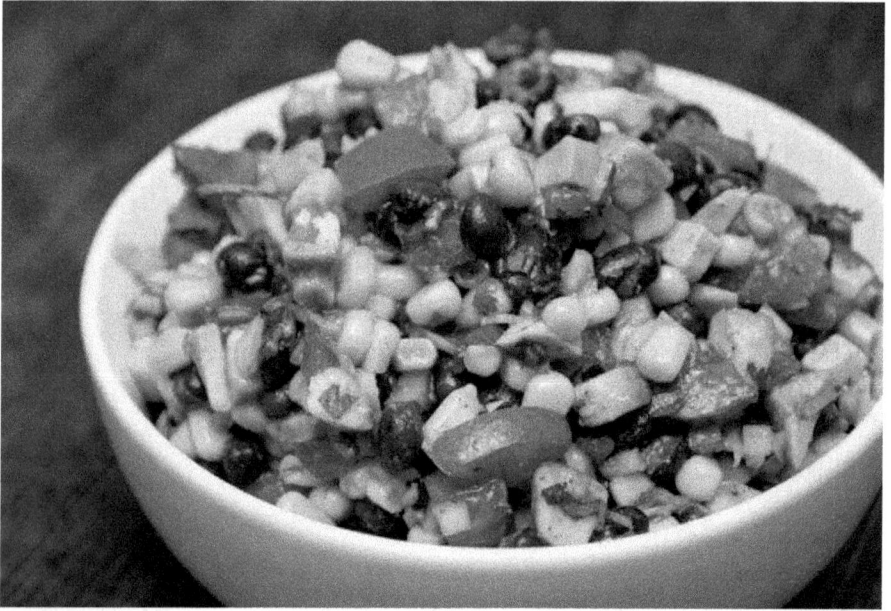

Mediterranean Turkey Bowls

Total time: 45 minutes
Servings: 4

Ingredients:

½ Medium cucumber
1 Bottle cucumber ranch dressing
½ Cup black olives
1 tbsp Dried basil
1 tsp Dried dill
2 tsp Dried marjoram
1 tbsp Dried oregano
1 tbsp Dried rosemary
4 ounces Feta
1 tsp Garlic powder
2 tbsp Greek seasoning
1 Green bell pepper
3 Green onions
¼ tsp Ground black pepper
½ tsp Ground thyme
1 pound Ground turkey
1 Head romaine lettuce
1 tbsp. Olive oil
1 package Pita chips
1 tsp Salt

Directions:

1.Get this meal started by making the seasoning

2.The first step is done by combining all the Ingredients: in a jar with a lid cover and shake well to mix properly.

3.Place a skillet over medium heat and pour the olive oil into it

4.Add the ground turkey into the skillet and wait for the turkey to get cooked through.

5.Pour the seasons into the skillet with the turkey and stir to mix and coat the turkey

6.Switch or turn off the heat to and set the skillet aside.

7.Wash the romaine and get the romaine chopped up.

8.Properly Wash and dice the green onions, bell pepper, and cucumber into small-sized pieces.

9.To serve, dish a large handful of lettuce in an eating bowl or plate. Add green onion, bell pepper, cucumber, olives, and feta as toppings

10.Overstep 9, add a spoonful of turkey and as toppings, add pita chips.

11.Drizzle the cucumber ranch dressing over the top and serve immediately.

Mediterranean Lemon Chicken

Total time:65 minutes

Ingredients:

6 Chicken legs
2 tsp Dried oregano
¼ tsp Ground black pepper
1 Lemon
3 cloves Minced garlic
1 tbsp Olive oil
¼ tsp Salt

Directions:

1.Switch on your oven and preheat to 425 °F

2.Get a 9x13-inch baking dish

3.Peel off the lemon bark and slice into halves.

4.Squeeze out the lemon juice to fill about ¼ cup and add the peel to the juice also the oregano, garlic, oil, salt, and pepper.

5.Properly stir to mix well.

6.Peel off the skin of the chicken pieces to dispose of them

7.Use the lemon mixture to coat the pieces of the chicken and arrange side by side with proper space in-between

8.Make sure the bone-side is up in the baking dish with the lid or cover on

9.Transfer to the oven and bake for about 20 minutes.

10.Turn the chicken over to baste it.

11.Tune the heat down to about 400 °F or 205 ° C) and bake with the lid or cover off, basting the chicken every 10 minutes, three times to make 30minutes in total

12.Serve chicken hot with pan juices.

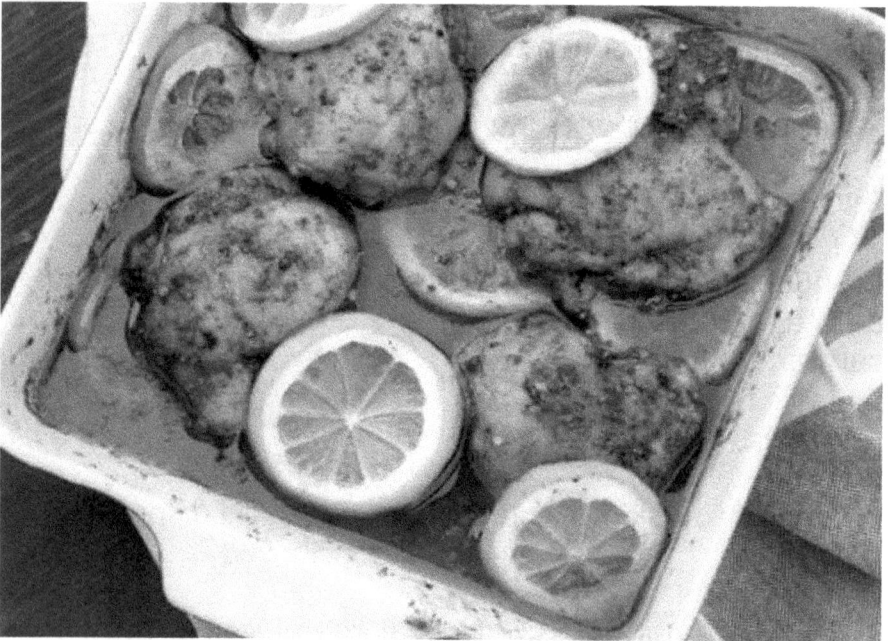

Chicken with Olives & Capers

Total time:65 minutes
Servings: 4

Ingredients:

2 tbsp Drained nonpareil capers
2 tbsp Extra-virgin olive oil
Freshly ground pepper
1 Lemon juice
1 cup Mixed pitted olives
2 pounds Organic chicken thighs (4large or 8 small)pounds
Salt
1 Wedge-shaped lemon

Directions:

1.Ensure oven is preheated to about 400°F

2.Place a rack in the middle section of the oven.

3.Put chicken unto a baking dish with the side up.

4.Spread the lemon wedges, olives, and capers on top of the chicken.

5.Juice up the chicken with lemon juice and olive oil generously with sprinkles of salt and pepper.

6.Transfer chicken with the mixtures and coatings into the oven to bake until chicken turns golden, should be achieved in about 25-30 minutes or till 165 °F

7.Serve while hot.

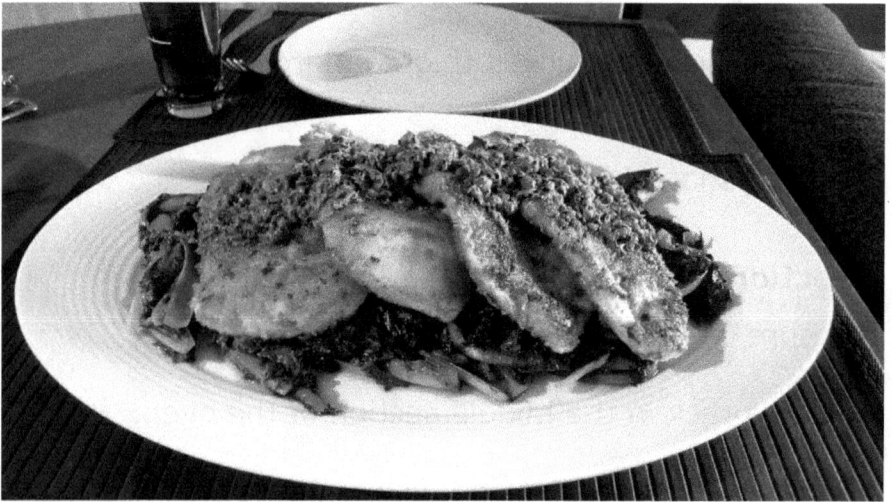

Slow Cooker Mediterranean Whole Chicken

Total time:8 hours 4
Servings: 4

Ingredients:

1 tbsp Ground oregano
1 tsp Ground pepper
1 tsp Kosher salt
2 tbsp Lemon juice
2 tsp Lemon zest
3 cloves Minced garlic cloves
1 tbsp Olive oil
4 pounds whole Chicken

Directions:

1.Get a small bowl to mix oregano, olive oil, lemon zest, garlic cloves, salt, and pepper.

2.Then take about 4 or 5 foil sheets and roll into balls to place at the bottom of the slowly burning cooker to serve as stands

3.Position the chicken on top of the balls, so the chicken does not stick to the cooker's bottom.

4.Coat the chicken with the readymade seasoning mix

5.Generously pour the lemon juice all over the chicken.

6.Cover up chicken and cook over low heat for about 8 hours or over high heat for about 4 hours

7.Wait for the time-lapse of till chicken is cooked through

8.Serve whole chicken combined with veggies and rice.

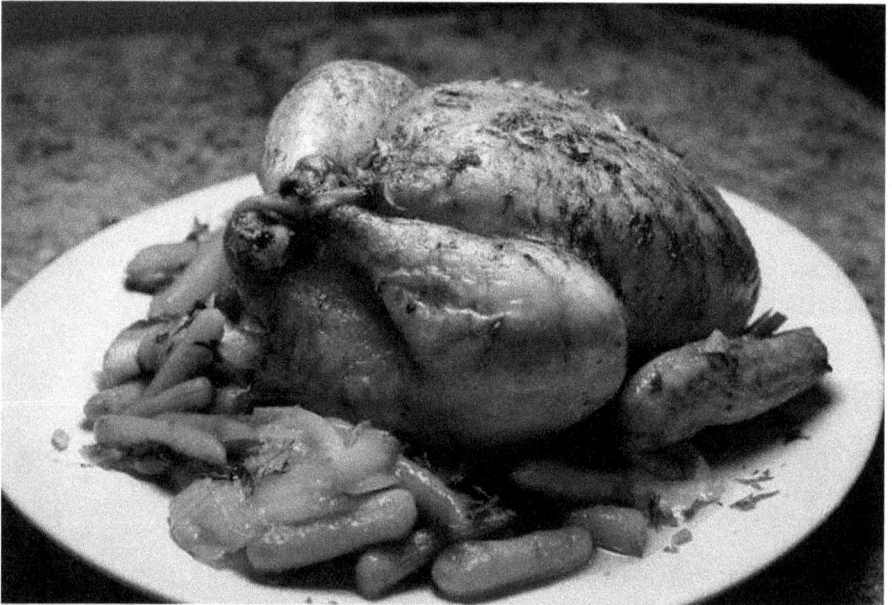

Oh-So Delicious Mediterranean Drumsticks

Total time:45 minutes
Servings:6

Ingredients:

¼ cup Barbeque sauce (any variety)
12 Chicken drumsticks (about 4¼ pounds)
½ cup Cooking wine
5 cloves Garlic
¼ cup Mustard

Directions:

1.Start by mixing the Ingredients:, wine, barbeque sauce, mustard and garlic in a large Ziplock bag.

2.Put drumsticks into the bag and, by chance marinate in the refrigerator for several hours

3.Get a large baking pan ready

4.Empty contents of the ziplock bag into the baking pan, ensuring the drumsticks all lie in a single layer.

5.Leave uncovered

6.Transfer to the oven and bake for 40 minutes at 400°F or till drumstick turns brown on both sides.

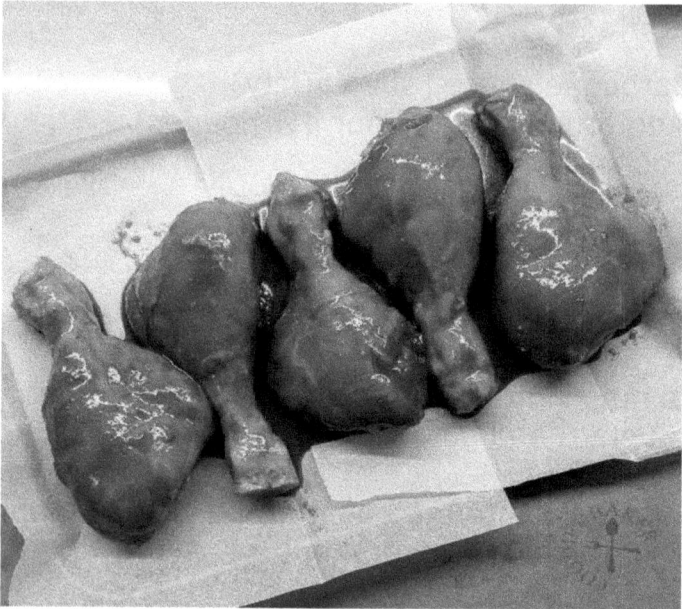

Greek Chicken Meal Prep Bowls

Total time:90 minutes
Servings: 5

Ingredients:

1 cup brown rice
½ pounds halves of cherry tomatoes

For the chicken:

2 pounds Chicken breasts (skinless and boneless)

1 tbsp Dried oregano

Freshly ground black pepper
Kosher salt
1 Lemon (juice)
3 cloves Minced garlic
¼ cup Olive oil
1 tbsp Red wine vinegar

For the cucumber salad:

½ tsp Dried oregano
1 Lemon(juice)
2 tbsp Olive oil
2 Peeled and sliced English cucumbers
2 cloves Pressed garlic
1 tbsp Red wine vinegar
½ cup Thinly sliced red onion

For the tzatziki sauce:

1 tbsp Chopped fresh dill
1 tsp Chopped fresh mint (optional)

1 Finely diced English cucumber
Freshly ground black pepper
1 tbsp Freshly squeezed lemon juice
Kosher salt
1 tsp Lemon zest
2 tbsp Olive oil
1 cup Plain Greek yogurt
2 cloves Pressed garlic

Directions:

1.Put chicken, ¼ cup olive oil, garlic, lemon juice, red wine vinegar and oregano in a Ziploc bag, shake properly to mix the Ingredients:

2.Then, season with salt and pepper to improve the taste

3.Marinate for about 20 minutes at the least and maximum of 1 hour, flipping over the bag occasionally.

4.Get the chickendrained offf the marinade, to dispose of the marinade

5.Using a large skillet, heat 2 tablespoons of olive oil over medium to high heat.

6.Put the chicken into the skillet and allow it to cook through for about 3-4 minute on each side.

7.Allow chicken to cool before dicing to small pieces.

8.To make the cucumber sala.d

9.Bring together cucumbers, onion, lemon, juice, olive oil, red wine vinegar,garlic, , and oregano into a small bowl and set aside

10.To make the tzatziki sauce

11.Bring together Greek yogurt, cucumber, garlic, dill, lemon juice, lemonzest, , and mint into a small bowl and season, adding salt and pepper to improve taste

12.Drizzle with olive oil and place in the fridge for about 10 minutes at the least, letting the flavors meld, then set apart.

13.Fill a large saucepan and 2 cups of water to cook rice according to package Directions:sand also set aside.

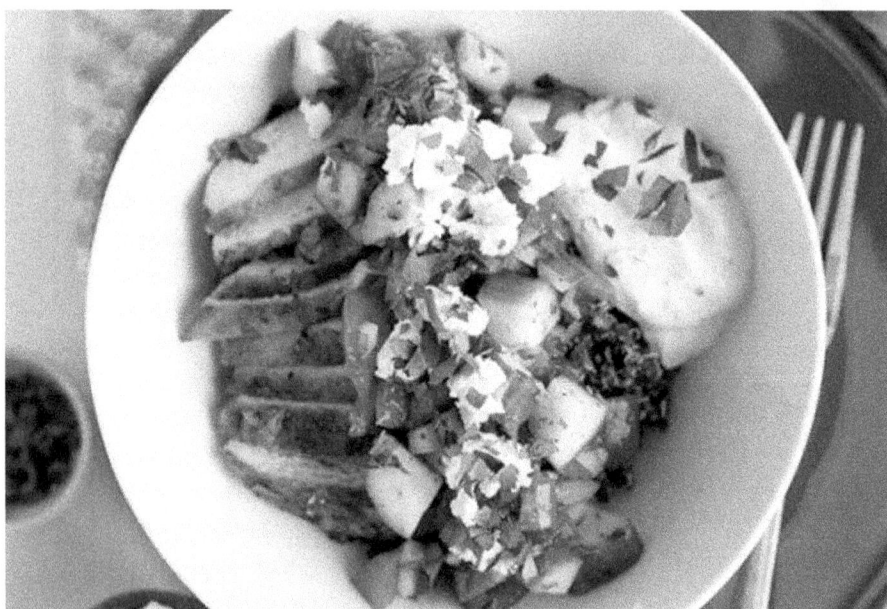

Chocolate and Date Smoothie

Preparation Time: 10 minutes
Cooking Time: 0 minutes
Servings: 2

Ingredients:

Medjool dates, pitted tbsp.
cacao powder tbsp. flaxseed
1 tbsp. almond butter
1 tsp vanilla extract
¼ tsp ground cinnamon
1½ cups almond milk, unsweetened ice cubes

Directions:

1.Add all ingredients in a high-power blender and pulse until smooth.

2.Pour into two glasses and serve immediately.

3.It can be stored in the fridge in a proper container up to 3 days.

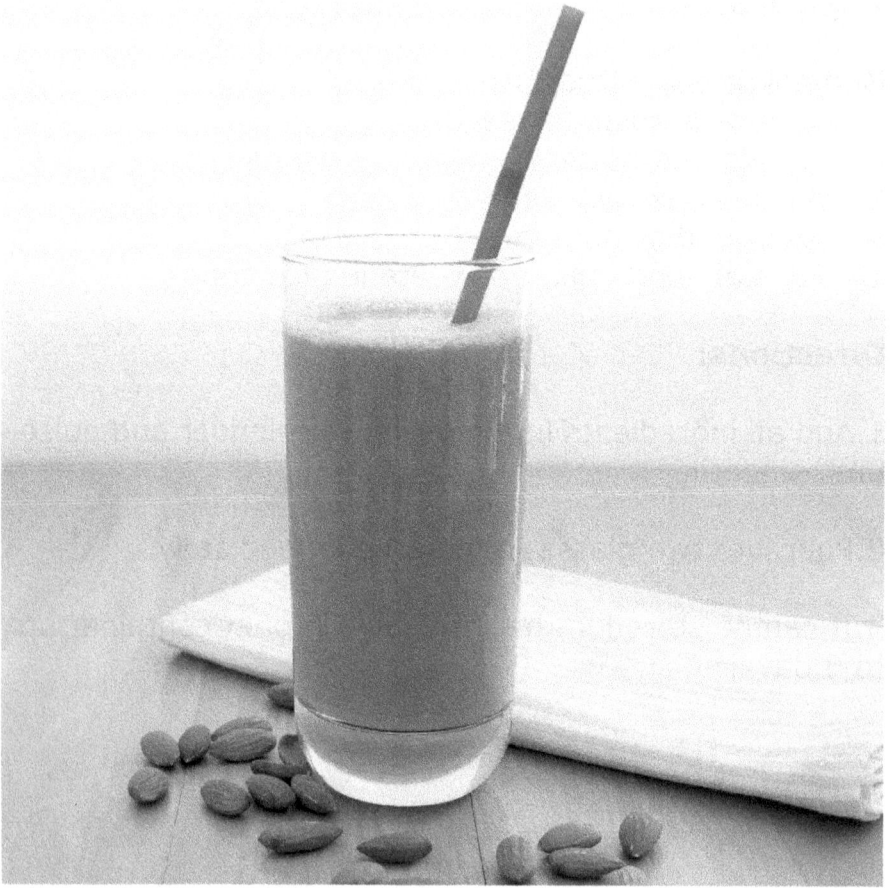

Cheese Baby Potatoes

Preparation Time: 10 minutes

Cooking Time: 20 minutes
Servings: 2

Ingredients:

4 baby potatoes
2 oz Cheddar cheese, shredded
¼ tsp. garlic powder
1 tsp. avocado oil

Directions:

1.Cut the baby potatoes into halves and sprinkle with garlic powder and avocado oil.

2.Bake the potatoes for 10 minutes at 365F.

3.Then top them with Cheddar cheese and bake for 10 minutes more.

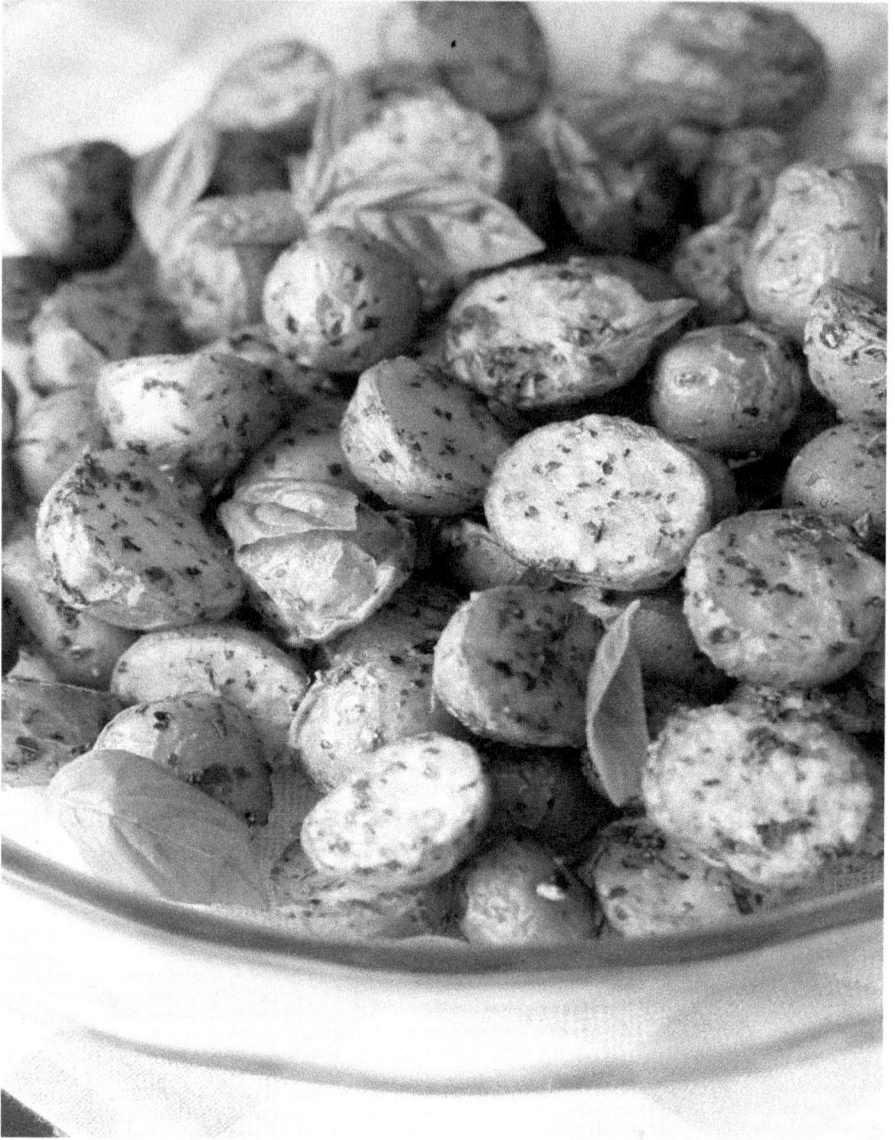

Tuna Paste

Preparation Time: 5 minutes
Cooking Time: 0 minutes
Servings: 6

Ingredients:

7 oz tuna, canned
2 tbsp. cream cheese
1 tbsp. chives, chopped

Directions:

1.Put all ingredients in the bowl and stir well with the help of the fork.

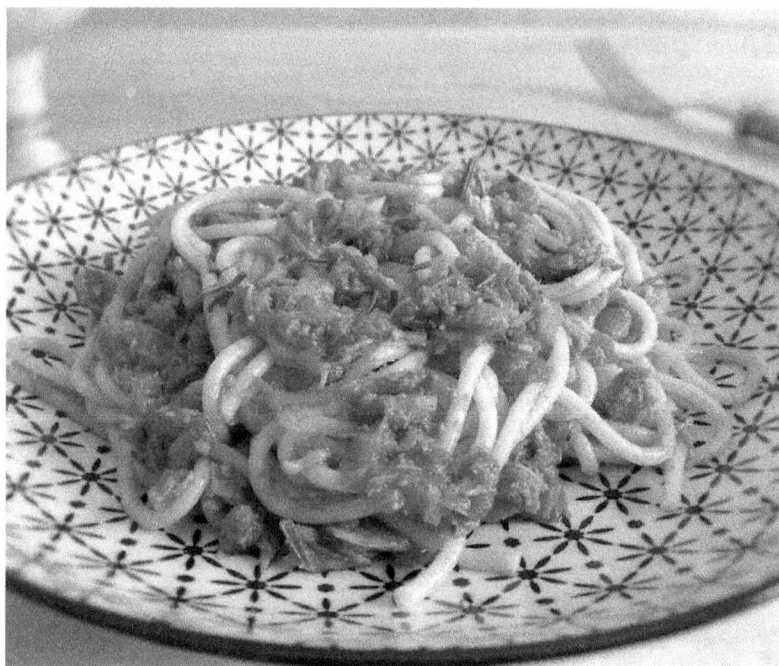

Zucchini Chips

Preparation Time: 5 minutes

Cooking Time: 12 minutes
Servings: 10

Ingredients:

2 zucchinis, thinly sliced
1 oz Parmesan, grated

Directions:

1.Line the baking tray with baking paper.

2.Put the zucchini in the tray in one layer and top with Parmesan.

3.Bake the chips for 12 minutes at 375F.

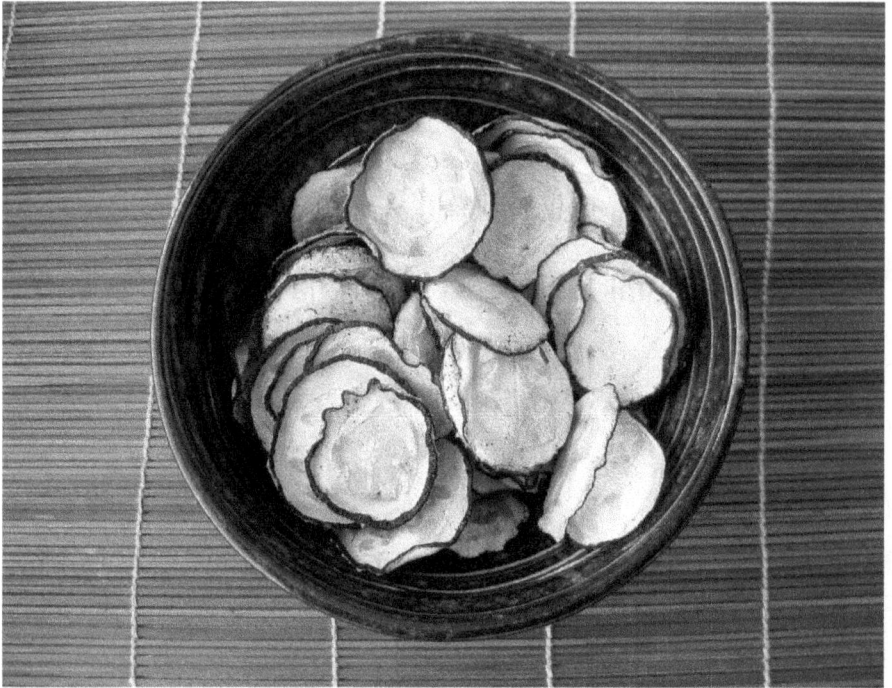

Crunchy Chickpeas

Preparation Time: 5 minutes
Cooking Time: 10 minutes
Servings: 2

Ingredients:

¼ cup chickpeas, canned
1 tbsp. avocado oil
1 tsp. ground paprika

Directions:

1.Line the baking tray with baking paper.

2.Mix up chickpeas with ground paprika and avocado oil and transfer the mixture in the tray. Flatten it gently.

3.Bake the chickpeas for 10 minutes at 400F. Stir them every 2 minutes.

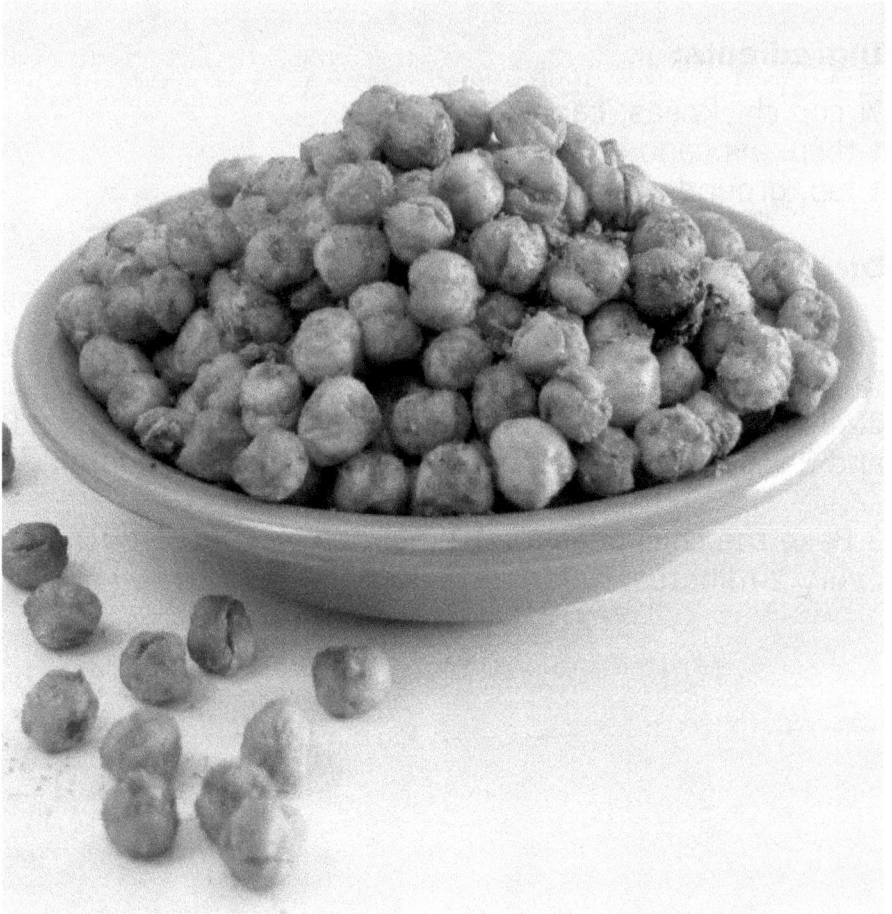

Stuffed Dates

Preparation Time: 5 minutes
Cooking Time: 0 minutes
Servings: 4

Ingredients:
4 dates, pitted
4 walnuts

Directions:

1.Fill the dates with walnuts.

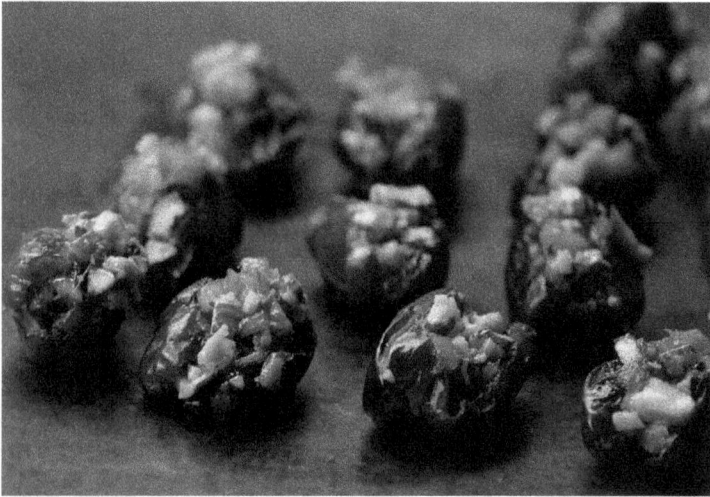

Almond Gazpacho

Preparation Time: 15 minutes
Cooking Time: 0 minutes
Servings: 4

Ingredients:

½ cup almonds
1 cup cucumbers, chopped
½ tsp. minced garlic
3 oz water, warm
2 oz chives, chopped
1 tbsp. sunflower oil
¼ cup fresh dill, chopped
¼ cup plain yogurt

Directions:

1.Put all ingredients in the blender and blend until smooth.

2.Cool the cooked gazpacho in the fridge for 10-15 minutes.

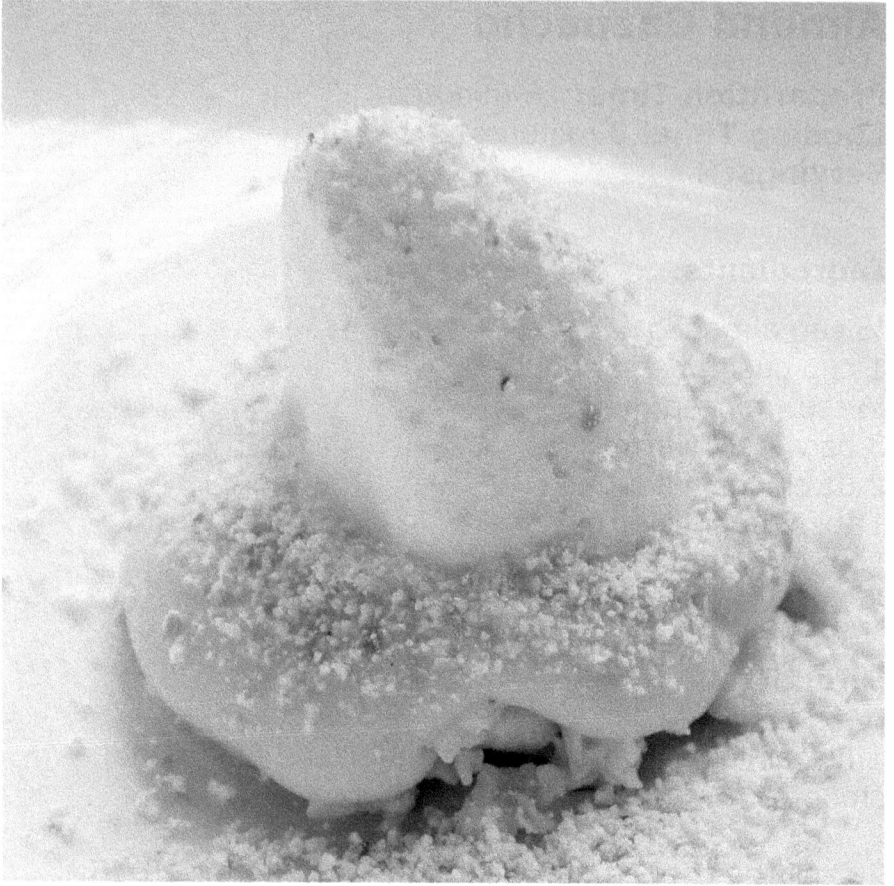

Turkey Chowder

Preparation Time: 5 minutes
Cooking Time: 20 minutes
Servings: 2

Ingredients:

½ cup ground turkey
¼ cup leek, chopped
1 tsp. dried rosemary
1 cup of water
1 cup plain yogurt
1 tsp. olive oil

Directions:

1.Roast the ground turkey with olive oil in the pan for 10 minutes. Stir well.

2.Then add all remaining ingredients and close the lid.

3.Cook the chowder for 10 minutes more on the medium heat.

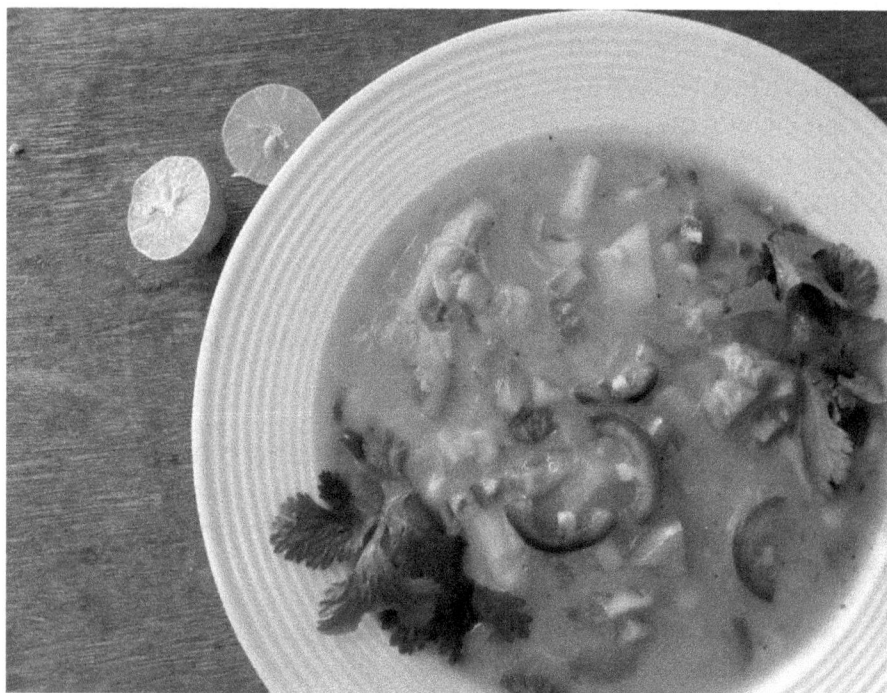

Blueberry & Kale Smoothie

Preparation Time: 10 minutes
Cooking Time: 0 minutes
Servings: 2

Ingredients:
cups frozen blueberries
cups fresh kale leaves Medjool dates, pitted
1 tbsp. chia seeds
1 ½-inch piece fresh ginger, peeled and chopped
1½ cups almond milk, unsweetened

Directions:

1.Add all ingredients in a high-power blender and pulse until smooth.

2.Pour the smoothie into two glasses and serve immediately.

3.It can be stored in the fridge in a proper container up to 3 days.

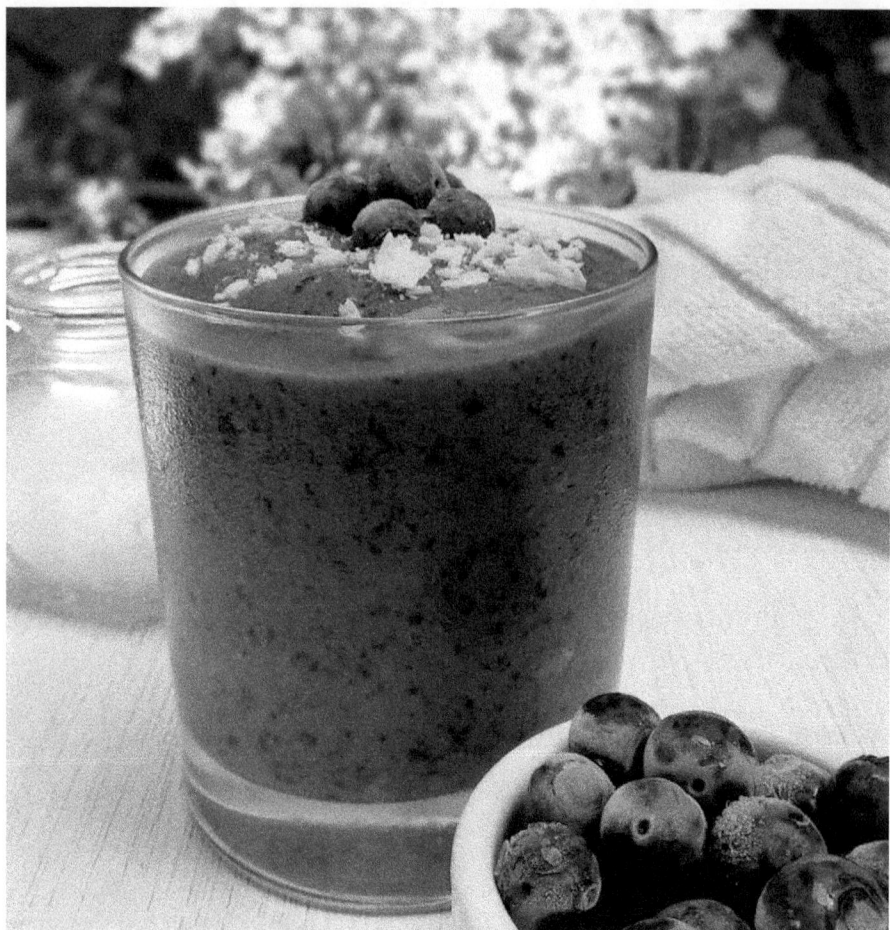

Strawberry & Beet Smoothie

Preparation Time: 10 minutes
Cooking Time: 0 minutes
Servings: 2

Ingredients:

cups frozen strawberries, pitted and chopped
2/3 cup frozen beets, chopped
1 ½-inch piece ginger, chopped
1 ½-inch piece fresh turmeric, chopped (or 1 tsp turmeric powder)
½ cup fresh orange juice
1 cup almond milk, unsweetened

Directions:

1.Add all ingredients in a high-power blender and pulse until smooth.

2.Pour the smoothie into two glasses and serve immediately.

3.It can be stored in the fridge in a proper container up to 3 days.

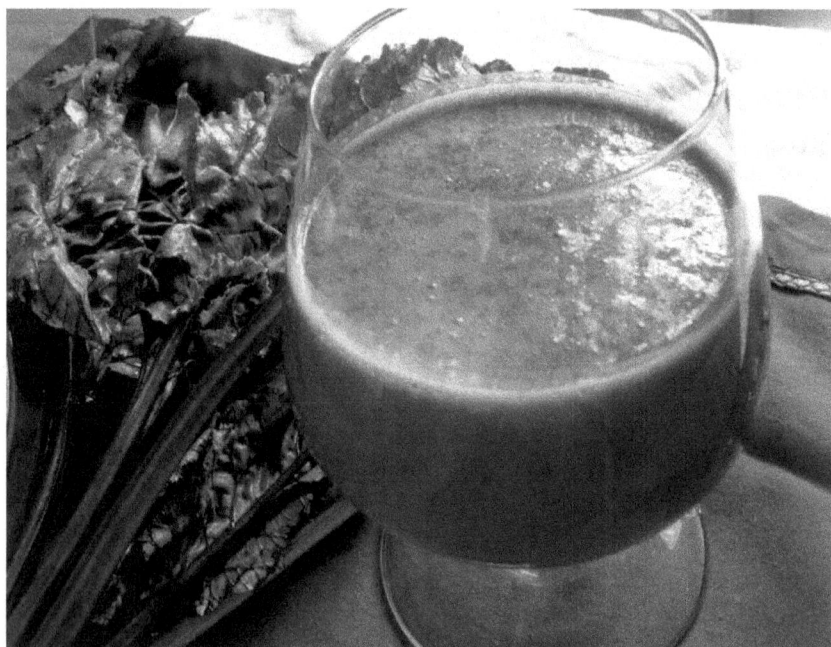

Corn and Zucchini Fritters

Preparation time: 15 minutes
Cooking time: 4 minutes
Servings: 12

Ingredients:

2 cups all-purpose flour
1 tbsp baking powder
½ tsp cumin
½ cups sugar
½ tsp salt
2 eggs, beaten
1 cup milk
¼ cup melted butter
2cups grated zucchini
1 ½ cups fresh corn
Cheddar cheese finely shredded
1 cup oil for frying

Directions:

1.In a big cup, mix flour and baking powder add cumin, sugar with salt and pepper.

2.In a shallow cup, mix the eggs and milk with butter together. Whisk the wet ingredients with the dry ingredients. Finally, Stir in courgette, corn, and cheese; blend well.

3.Heat some oil in a steel skillet over low heat. Add the spoonful of the batter to the hot liquid. Fry until brown. Turn the tongs once. Drop on the paper towels.

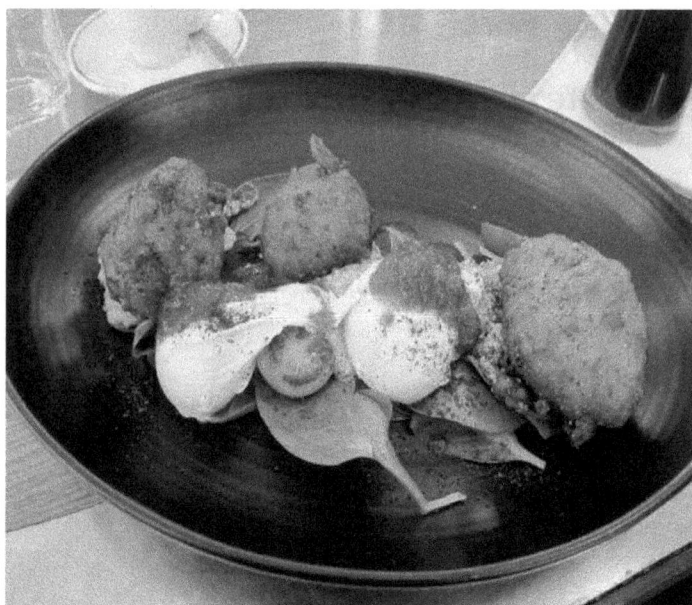

Grilled Aubergine Panini

Preparation time: 10 minutes
Cooking time: 25 minutes **Servings:** 4

Ingredients:

2 tbsp Mayonnaise reduced-fat
2 tbsp Fresh basil sliced
2 tbsp Extra-virgin olive oil, separated
8 ounces Eggplant slices
Garlic salt ½ teaspoon
8 slices Whole-grain country bread
8 ounces Fresh mozzarella cheese
8 thin slices Roasted red peppers sliced jarred
⅓ cup Red onion, four pieces four thin slices

Directions:

1. Preheat grill to about medium-high flame.

2. In a shallow tub, mix mayonnaise and basil. Using one tablespoon of the oil, gently brush both the sides of the eggplant and then sprinkle each piece with garlic salt. Coat one side of every piece of bread using the residual one tablespoon of the oil.

3. Grill the eggplant now for about 6 minutes, turning its side with the spatula, covering with the cheese, and then proceeding to grill till the cheese gets melted. The eggplant is soft, around 4 minutes longer. Cook the bread upon this grill for about 1 to 2 minutes each foot.

4. To produce sandwiches: scatter the mayonnaise basil over four pieces of bread. Cover with cheesy eggplant,

red pepper, onion, and the remaining pieces of bread.
Break it in half, then serve hot.

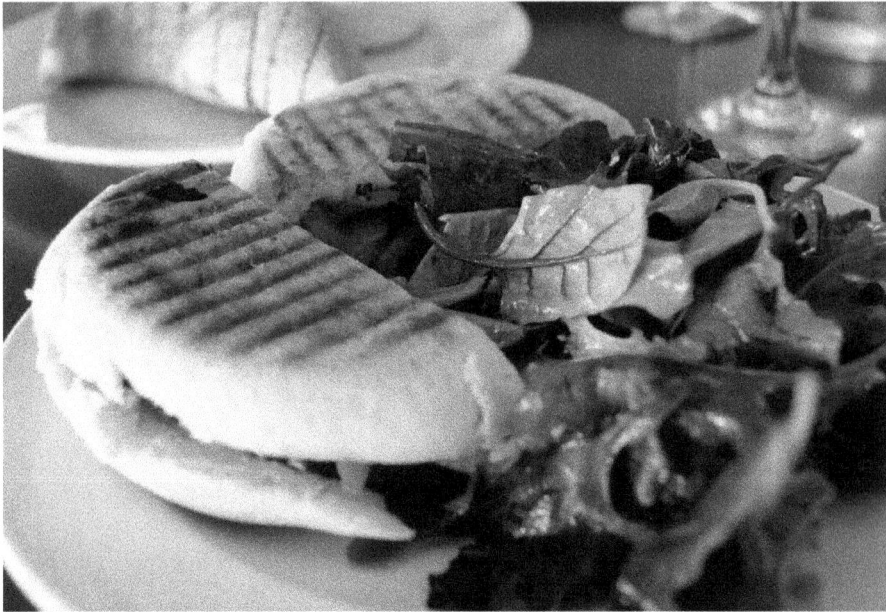

Roasted Vegetable Frittata

Preparation time:30 minutes
Cooking time:55 minutes
Servings: 4

Ingredients:

Orange sweet potato, skinned, cut into pieces (3cm),
350g Red capsicum, cut into pieces (3cm),
1 Red onions, cut into wedges
2 Zucchini, cut into pieces (3cm)
2 Olive oil as cooking spray
Eggs 6
1/3 cups Skim milk
100 g. Baby rocket
20 g. Parmesan cheese, shaved
¼ cup Walnuts, roughly sliced
1 tbsp Balsamic vinegar

Directions:

1.Preheat the oven to about 220°C. Oiled e a 6cm in-depth, 20cm wide, 8-cup square oven-safe bowl.

2.Line up a broad roasting pan with the baking paper. Put the sweet potatoes, capsicum, onions with zucchini in the tub. Spray the gasoline. Place in a single thin layer and toast for about 30 minutes until it becomes golden and soft.

3.Spread the vegetables on the base of the prepared bowl. Reduce oven to a temperature of 190°C. Mix the eggs, the milk as well as the pepper together in a cup. Pour the egg mixture over the vegetables, shake the dish gently to allow the egg to disperse to the base.

4.Bake the frittata for about 25 minutes or until the top is golden and the middle is set. Put aside for ten minutes. Break the mixture into 4 bits.

5.Place the rocket, the parmesan, and the walnuts in a dish. Toss to mix it. Divide the salad and the frittata onto the serving dishes.

6.Drop one teaspoon of vinegar into each salad. Now serve it

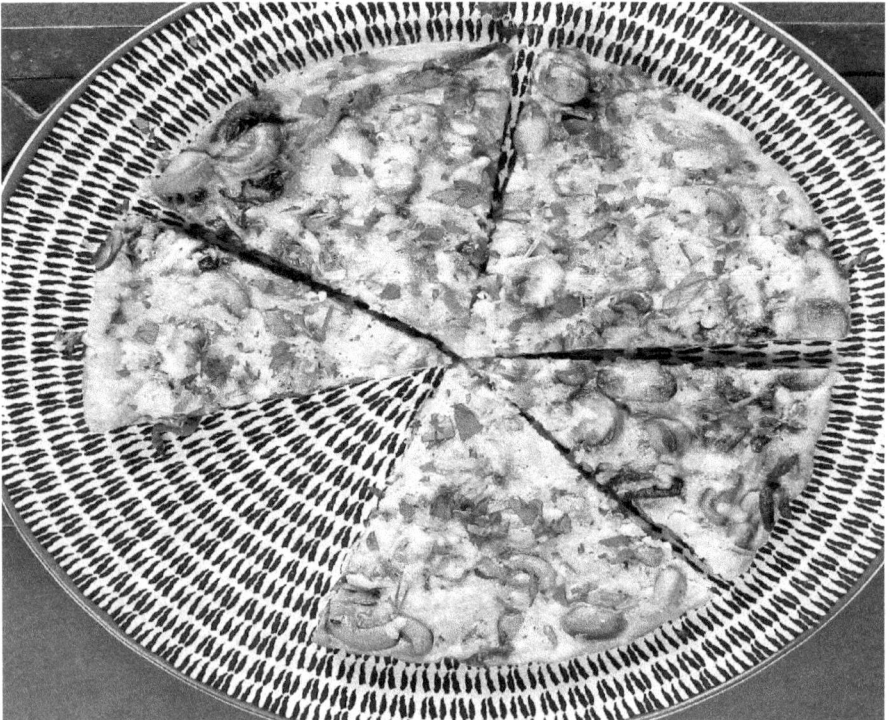

Pita Pockets

Preparation time: 3 hours
Cooking time: 10 minutes
Servings: 6

Ingredients:

2 cups Wheat Flour
2 tbsp Maida (All-purpose flour)
Active dry yeast, one packet
1 tsp Sugar
1 ¾ cup Milk or warm water
1 tbsp Oil
Salt, to taste

Directions:

1.Put all the products together. Preheat the oven to 400 degrees F. Dissolve the yeast with sugar in the warm milk or water and leave to stand for about 2-3 minutes till it becomes foamy.

2.Once the yeast is activated (foamy and bubbly), continue with the recipe. In case the yeast ceases to do so, kindly discard and start anew.

3.When the yeast has sprouted, mix all the ingredients inside a tub, add the yeast with oil then knead the dough.

4.Wrap the dough now with a moist cloth, then set aside for about 2-3 hours.

5.The dough would almost become double in size.

6.Divide the dough into similar balls.

7.Roll these in thick rings. Put the rolled dough over the baking sheet, then bake inside the oven for about 7-10 minutes till it becomes brown from the tip.

8.You'll see them buffing up shortly.

9.All puffed up.

10.Take them out from the oven, then let them cool down. Now serve the Pita bread pockets.

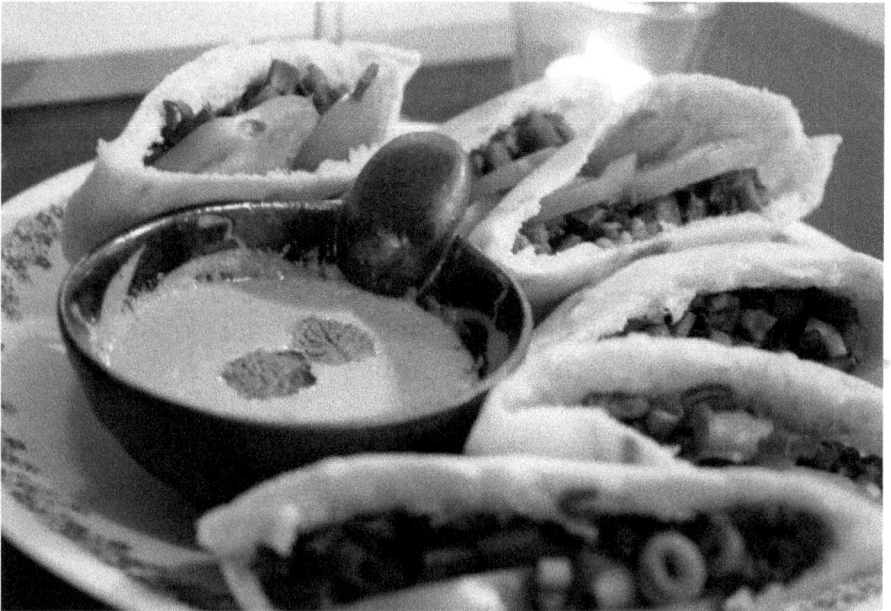

Chicken Guacamole Wraps

Preparation time:5 minutes
Cooking time:5 minutes
Servings: 4

Ingredients:

2 tbsp Fresh lime juice
¼ tsp Salt
Peeled avocado, one ripe
½ cup Seeded plum tomato chopped
Lettuce leaves, four green leaf
Flour tortillas (fat-free), 4 (8-inch)
2 cups Grilled Lemon-Herb Chicken (about 8 ounces)

Directions:

1.Put three ingredients first in a mixing saucepan; crush with a fork till smooth. Stir in the tomatoes.

2.Put one lettuce leaf around each tortilla; scatter around 1/4 cup of avocado paste over each lettuce leaf.

3.Cover each portion with 1/2 cup of Roasted Lemon-Herb Chicken. Now roll-up. Cover either in foil or parchment, then chill

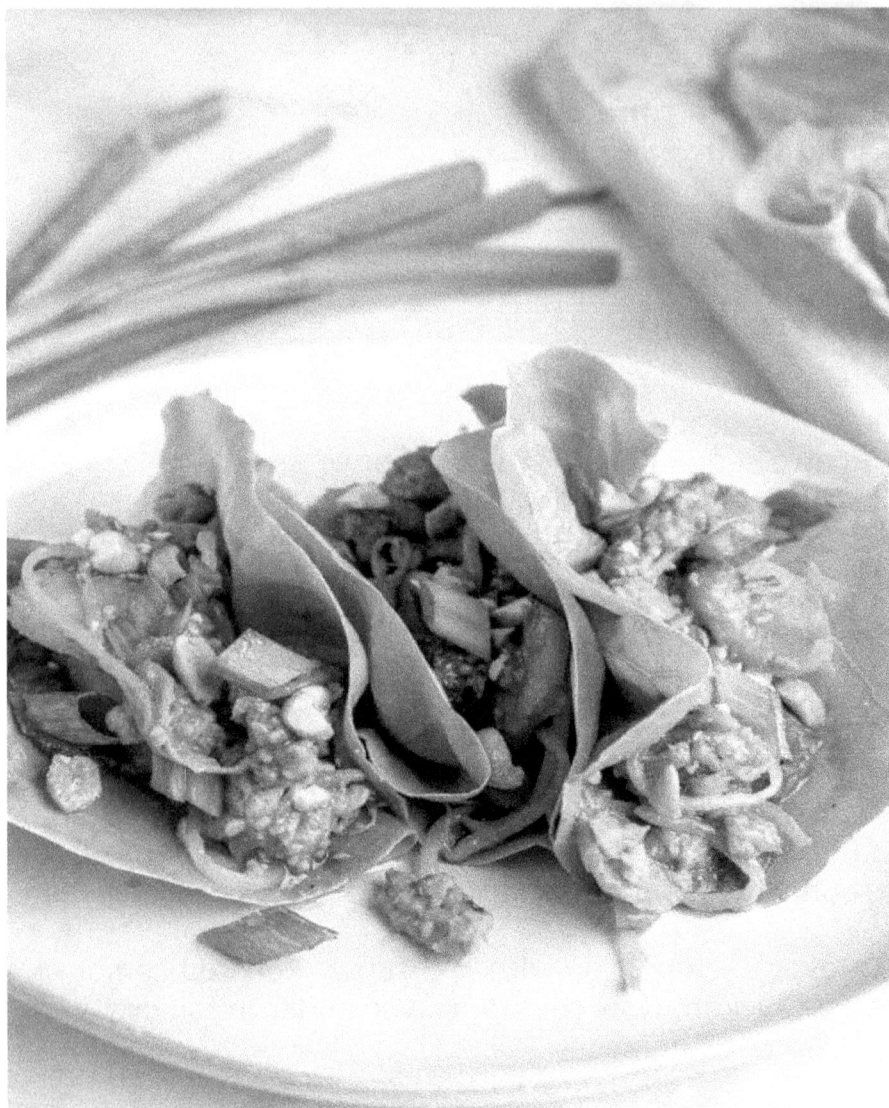

Italian Eggplant Salad

Preparation time: minutes
Cooking time: minutes
Servings: 4

Ingredients:

3 cups Cubed eggplant
2 tbsp White wine vinegar
1 clove Chopped garlic
1 Chopped onion
1/2 teaspoon oregano
3 tsp Olive oil
1/4 teaspoon black pepper
1 Chopped tomato

Directions:

1.Boil water in a saucepan. Add eggplant to boiling water in a saucepan.

2.Add eggplant in the boiling water and cook until tender (for about 10 minutes)

3.Drain the water and place onion and eggplant in a glass dish.

4.Mix vinegar, pepper, and garlic together.

5.Pour the mixture over eggplant and onion

6.Toss the mixture, eggplant, and onion together. Before serving, stir in oil.

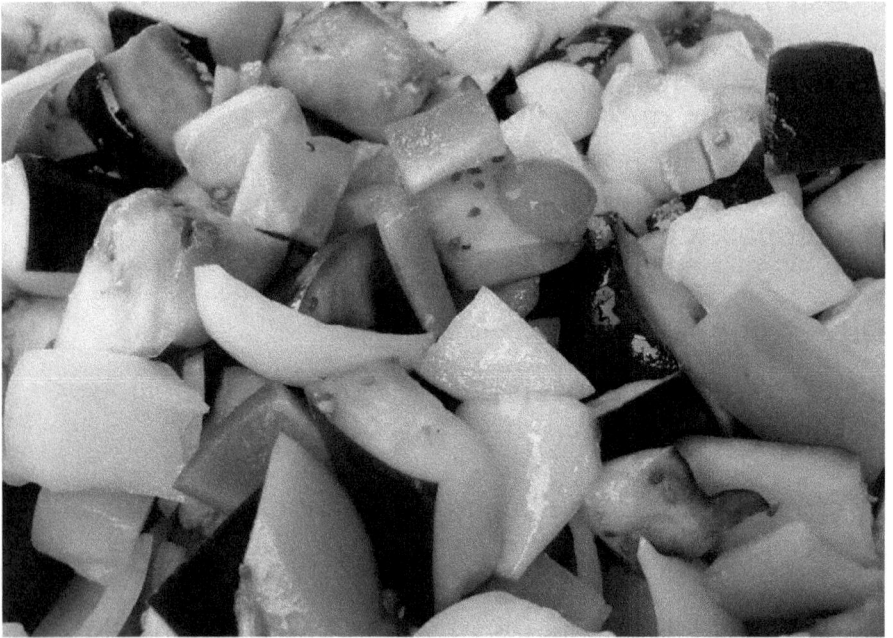

Cauliflower in Mustard Sauce

Preparation time: 10 minutes
Cooking time: 90 minutes
Servings: 4

Ingredients:

1 tsp Honey
2 tsp Dijon mustard
1 ½ tbsp White-wine vinegar
Dash black pepper
1 tbsp Olive oil
2 cups cauliflower flowerets

Directions:

1.Mix the mustard and honey in a bowl.

2. Add olive oil and vinegar to the bowl; Whisk

3.Season with black pepper. Set the bowl aside.

4.Boil water in a saucepan and add cauliflower to it.
Cook until tender.

5.Drain the cauliflower well and add it to the mixture
prepared earlier; Toss.

6.Give 30-45 minutes for the salad to cool down. Serve.

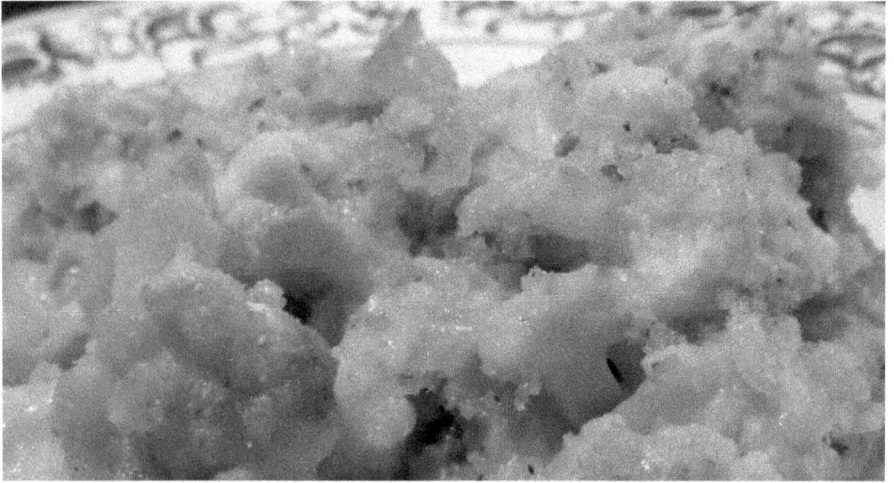

Pineapple Coleslaw

Preparation time: 5 minutes
Cooking time: 0 minute
Servings: 4

Ingredients:

2 cups shredded Cabbage
1/4 cup Miracle Whip
8 oz crushed pineapples
Pepper to taste
1/4 cup chopped onion

Directions:

1.Take a bowl. Add all the ingredients together; mix well.

2.Chill for 1 hour (at least). Serve

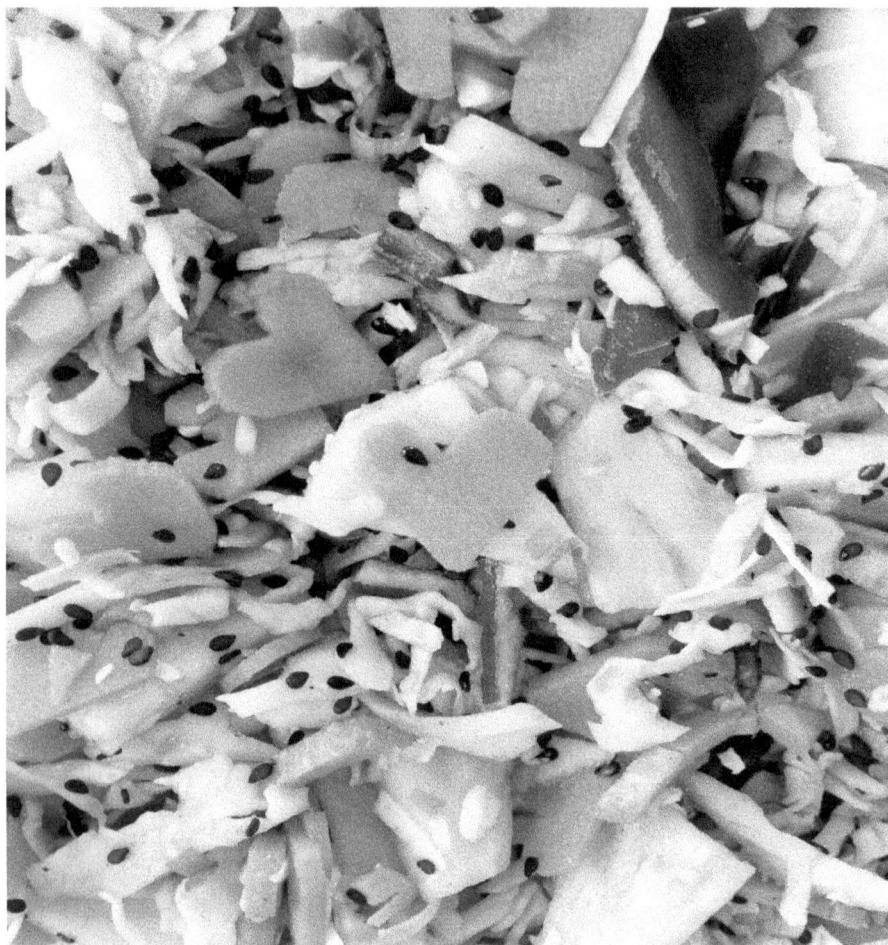

Basil Oil

Preparation time: 10 minutes
Cooking time: 10 minutes
Servings: 16

Ingredients:
1 cup Olive oil
1.5 cups Basil leaves

Directions:

1.Drain and Rinse the basil leaves.

2.Allow them to dry by patting them with a towel.

3.Add and Whirl basil leaves and olive oil in a blender or food processor (until leaves are finely chopped). Do not puree.

4.Take a 1 to 1 1/2-quart pan. Pour the mixture into the pan, heated medium.

5.Stir occasionally for 3-4 minutes (look for oil bubbles to gather around pan sides and when the thermometer reaches 165 degrees, remove the pan from the stove). To kill bacteria, make sure the oil is heated to the mentioned temperature.

6.Let the mixture cool (minimum one hour).

7.Take a fine wire strainer and line it with two layers of cheesecloth. Set the strainer over a small bowl.

8.Pour the earlier prepared oil mixture into the strainer.

9.Let the oil passes through. Afterward, keep gently pressing the basil to the remaining oil.

10.Discard the leftover basil in the filter.

For three months, store the oil in an airtight container (refrigerate). Don't worry if the olive oil solidifies when chilled. It will quickly liquefy when you bring it back to room temperature. (You can serve the oil right-away as well)

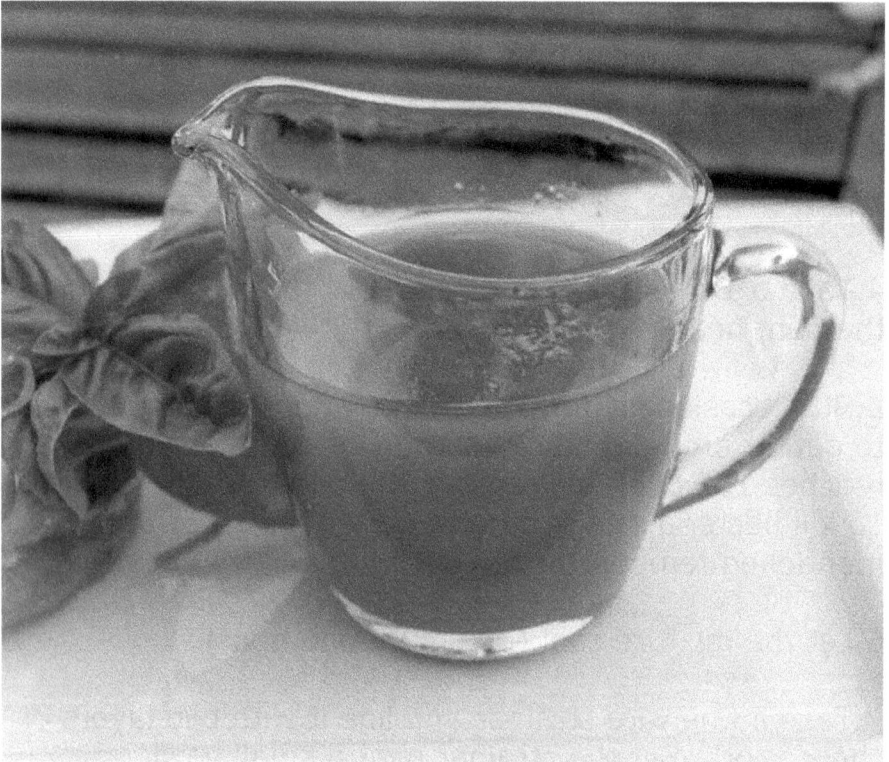

Black Eyed Peas

Preparation time: 2 minutes
Cooking time: 80 minutes
Servings: 12

Ingredients:

2 cups dried Black-eyed peas
5 cloves chopped Garlic 12 oz Smoked turkey
3 ½ cups Water
1 chopped Onion
1 pinch Cayenne pepper
1/2 tsp Ginger
1 cup diced Celery
1/2 tsp thyme
1/2 tsp Curry powder

Directions:

1.Take a large bowl. Add black-eyed peas. Pour water over them (just enough to cover the peas by about 4 inches). Cover the bowl and let soak overnight (or at least six hours).

2.Rinse the peas under cold water; Drain.

3.Take a large pot; add all the remaining ingredients and black-eyed peas to the pot.

4.Bring to boil. After the first boil, reduce heat to low.

5.Cook until peas are tender (covered with a lid) for about 1 hour.Stir occasionally.

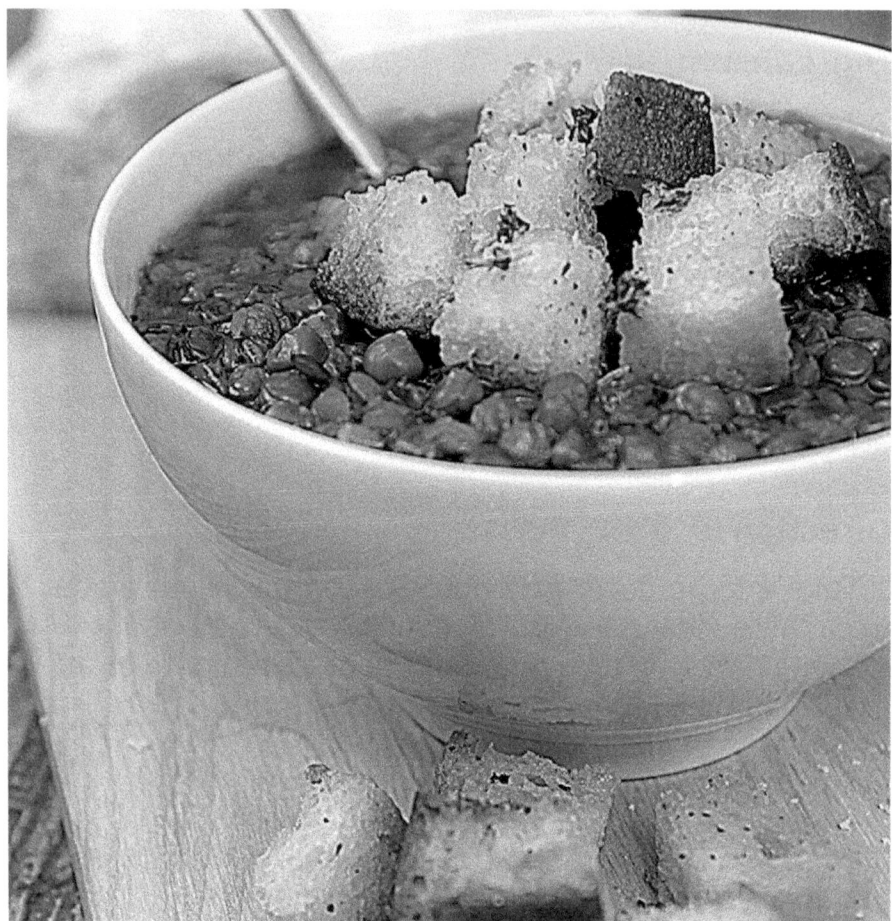

Blasted Brussel Sprouts

Preparation time: 8 minutes
Cooking time: 20 minutes
Servings: 2-3

Ingredients:
3 tbsp Grated Parmesan Cheese
2 cups Brussels Sprouts
1/4 cup Fruit or herb-flavored vinegar
2 tbsp Olive oil

Directions:

1.Preheat oven at 450 degrees.

2.Firstly, clean the old leaves off. Cut all the larger sprouts in half. Leave all the smaller sprouts whole.

3.Add olive oil; toss.

4.Put an oiled baking sheet (lightly oiled) on.

5.Roast for a while (about 10 minutes) until the sprouts are tender enough to be pierced using a fork.

6.Take out of the oven. Sprinkle with and Parmesan cheese and fruit vinegar.

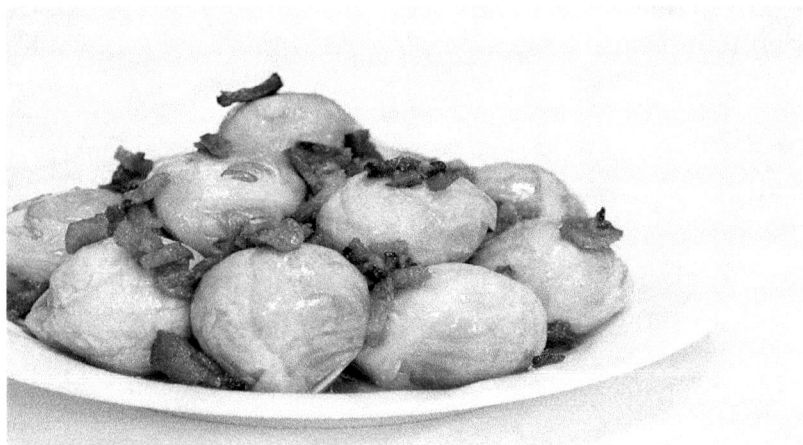

Roasted Tomatillo Salsa

Preparation time: 10 minutes
Cooking time: 10 minutes
Servings: 8

Ingredients:
1 lb Tomatillos
1 Head garlic
¼ cup Water
1 bunch Cilantro
3 Jalapenos Lime juice to taste

Directions:

1.Take tomatillos, cut them in half.

2.Take an Oil baking sheet. Spread tomatillos, jalapenos, and garlic, on it. Coat with oil; toss.

3.Turn the tomatillos brown (for about 10-15 minutes). Remove from heat (oven).

4.Take a food processor, blend all the ingredients, including tomatillos (until everything is smooth). Serve with corn chips over burritos, tacos, or enchiladasors.

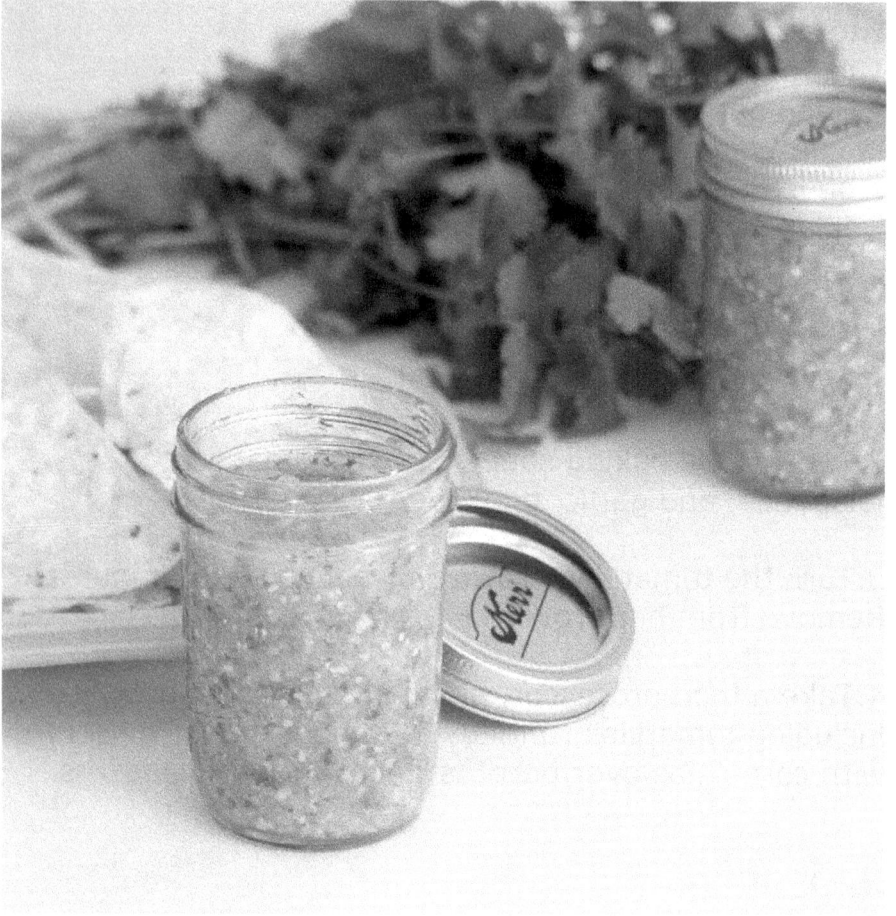

Pico de Gallo

Preparation time: 15 minutes
Cooking time: 0 minute
Servings: 2-3

Ingredients:

3 chopped bell Peppers
1 cup Jicama
Salt to taste
5 Garlic cloves
1 tbsp Sugar
½ chopped Purple onion To taste
Lime Juice

Directions:

1.Take a Food processor; Add all ingredients in it. Pulse and enjoy your salsa!

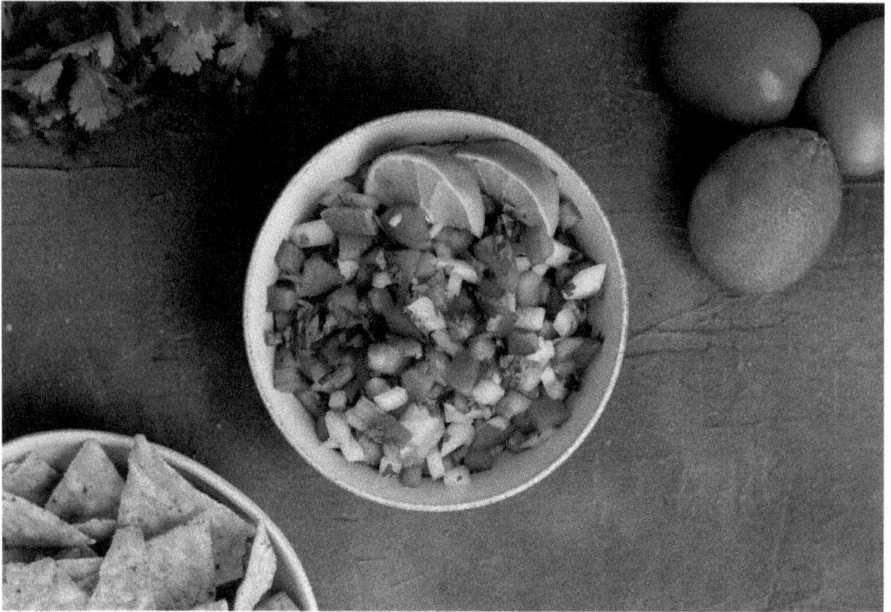

Beans and Ham

Preparation time: 10 minutes
Cooking time: 50 minutes
Servings: 6

Ingredients:

1/2 cup ham
1 cup White rice
1 cup lima beans
4 Garlic cloves
1.5 cups diced Onion
2 tbsp Cider vinegar
1 tbsp Honey
3 tbsp Oil
2 Jalapeno peppers
½ tsp Smoked paprika
32 oz Chicken broth
½ tsp Ground pepper
¼ tsp Salt

Directions:

1.Add rice and beans in a pressure cooker with low sodium chicken broth and 2 cups water.

2.Cook as per instructions of the pressure cooker (about 45 minutes for un-soaked and dry beans. Then 20 minutes at pressure. Then go for natural release).

3.Set the beans aside. Chop garlic and onions and sauté in oil. Set Aside.

4.Take a small bowl; combine the honey, vinegar, salt, paprika, jalapenos, and pepper to make your seasoning.

5.Add the seasoning mix, onion, and garlic to the rice and beans, along with the ham. Mix and Serve!

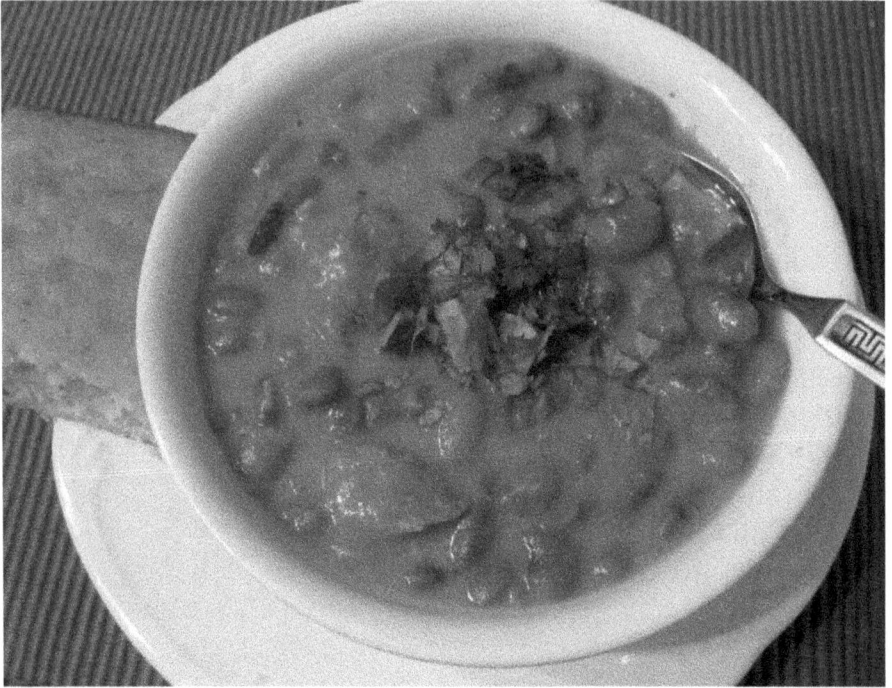

Green Pineapple Smoothie

Preparation Time: 5 minutes
Cooking Time: 0 minutes
Servings: 1

Ingredients:

1 cup spinach
1 apple
1 cup pineapple
1tsp. of flax seeds
½ cup filtered water

Directions:

1.Add all ingredients in a high-power blender and pulse until smooth.

2.Pour the smoothie into two glasses and serve immediately.

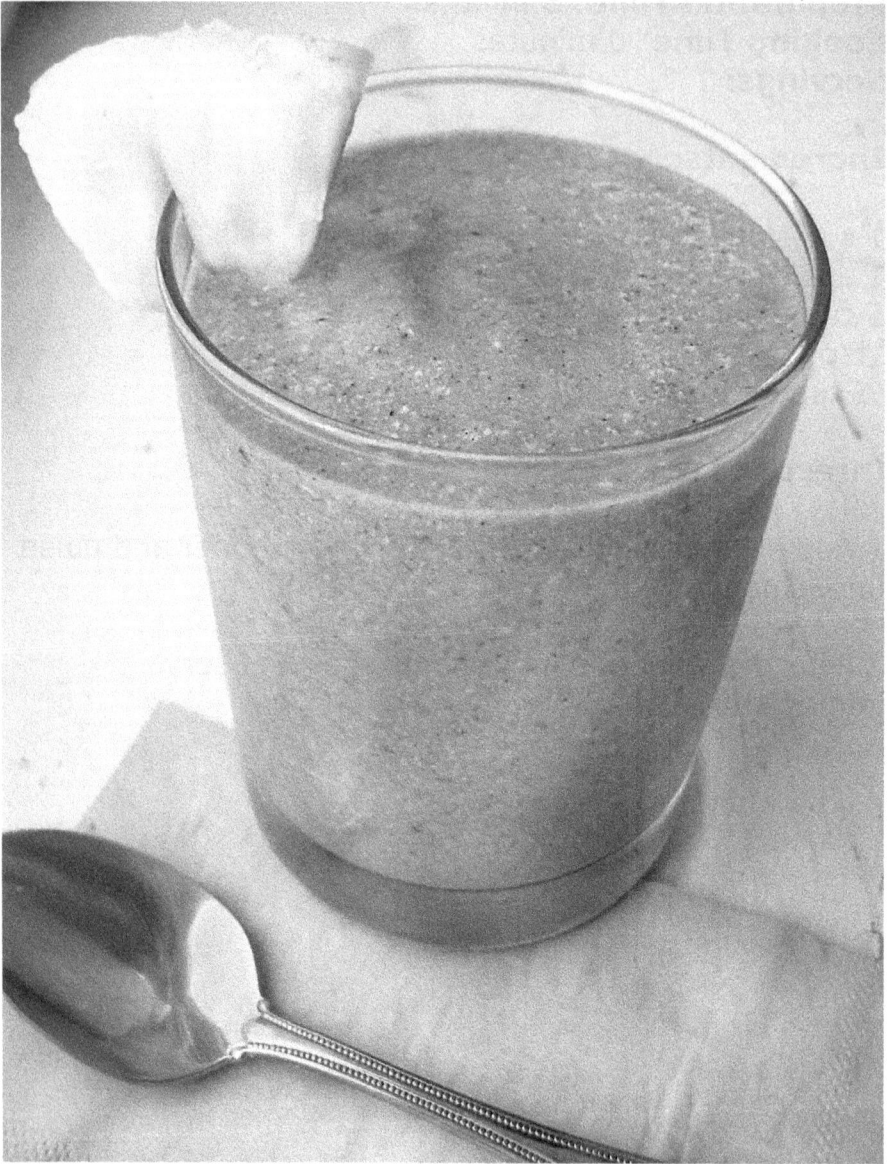

Spinach Smoothie

Preparation Time: 5 minutes
Cooking Time: 0 minutes
Servings: 1

Ingredients:

1 cup spinach
1 pear
½ bananas
½ cup almond milk, unsweetened

Directions:

1.Add all ingredients in a high-power blender and pulse until smooth.

2.Pour the smoothie into two glasses and serve immediately.

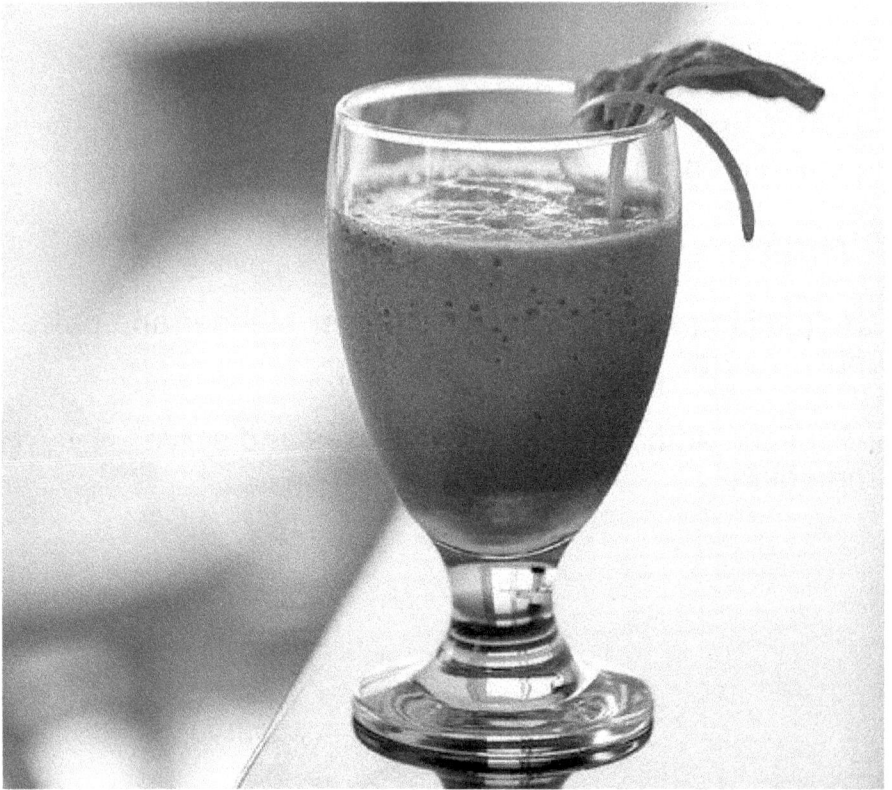

Kale Smoothie

Preparation Time: 5 minutes
Cooking Time: 0 minutes
Servings: 1

Ingredients:

1 cup kale
½ mango
½ banana
1 tbsp. chia seeds
¼ cup coconut milk, unsweetened
½ cup filtered water

Directions:

1.Add all ingredients in a high-power blender and pulse until smooth.

2.Pour the smoothie into two glasses and serve immediately

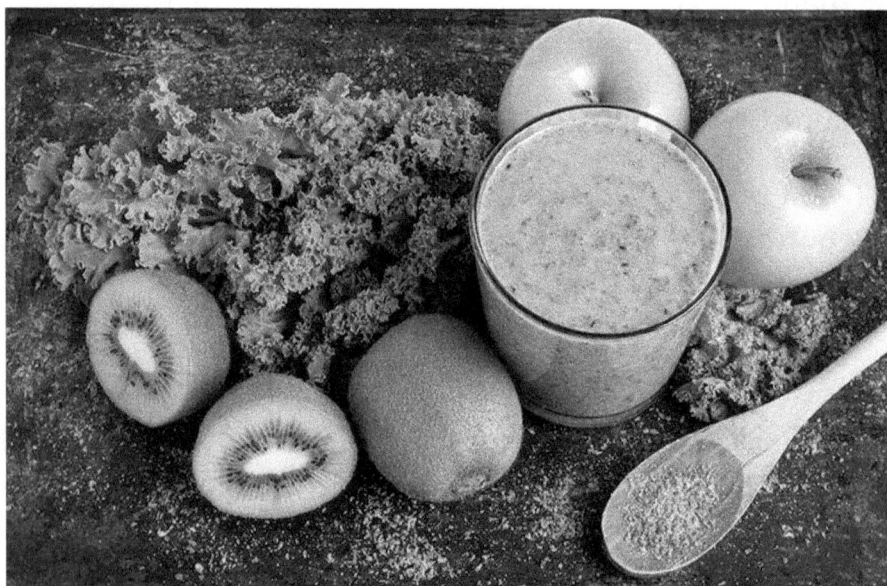

Avocado Smoothie

Preparation Time: 5 minutes
Cooking Time: 0 minutes
Servings: 1

Ingredients:

½ avocado
1 banana
1 cup spinach
1 tbsp. linseed
¼ cup almond milk, unsweetened
½ cup filtered water

Directions:

1.Add all ingredients in a high-power blender and pulse until smooth.

2.Pour the smoothie into two glasses and serve immediately

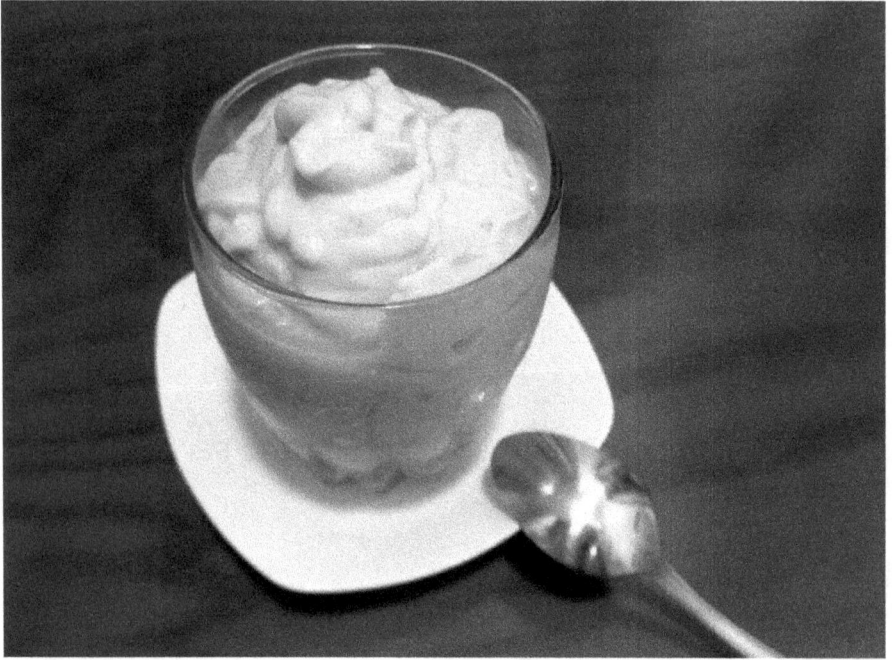

Lettuce Smoothie

Preparation Time: 5 minutes
Cooking Time: 0 minutes
Servings: 1

Ingredients:

½ small head of lettuce fresh plums, seeded
½ banana
1 tbsp. linseed
½ cucumber
½ cup almond milk, unsweetened

Directions:

1.Add all ingredients in a high-power blender and pulse until smooth.

2.Pour the smoothie into two glasses and serve immediately.

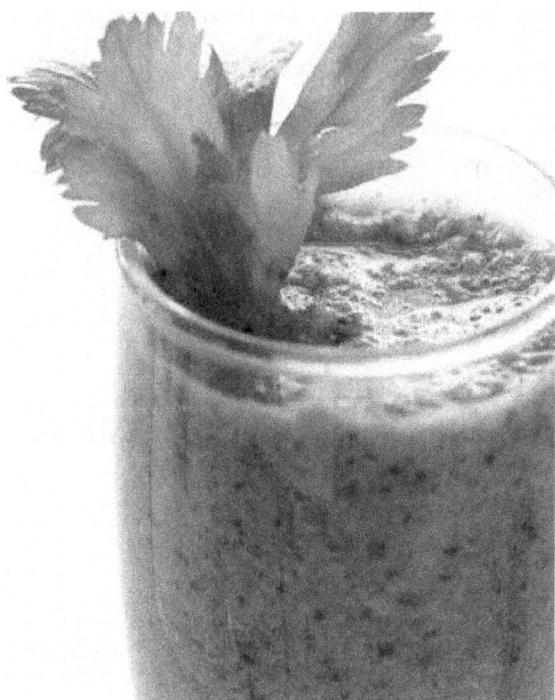

Strawberry, Mango and Yogurt Smoothie

Preparation Time: 5 minutes
Cooking Time: 0 minutes
Servings: 2

Ingredients:

1 mango, destoned, peeled, diced oz. strawberries
oz. yogurt
cups almond milk, unsweetened

Directions:

1.Add all ingredients in a high-power blender and pulse until smooth.

2.Pour the smoothie into two glasses and serve immediately.

3.It can be stored in the fridge in a proper container up to 3 days.

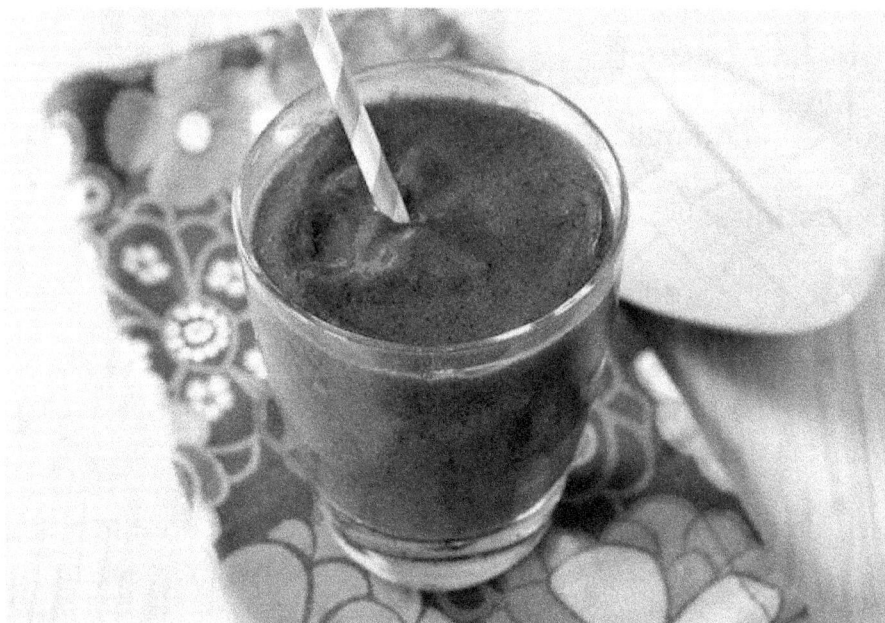

Berries Vanilla Protein Smoothie

Preparation Time: 5 minutes
Cooking Time: 0 minutes
Servings: 2

Ingredients:

oz. blackberries
oz. strawberries
oz. raspberries
scoops of vanilla protein powder
1 ½ cup almond milk, unsweetened

Directions:

1.Add all ingredients in a high-power blender and pulse until smooth.

2.Pour the smoothie into two glasses and serve immediately.

3.It can be stored in the fridge in a proper container up to 3 days.

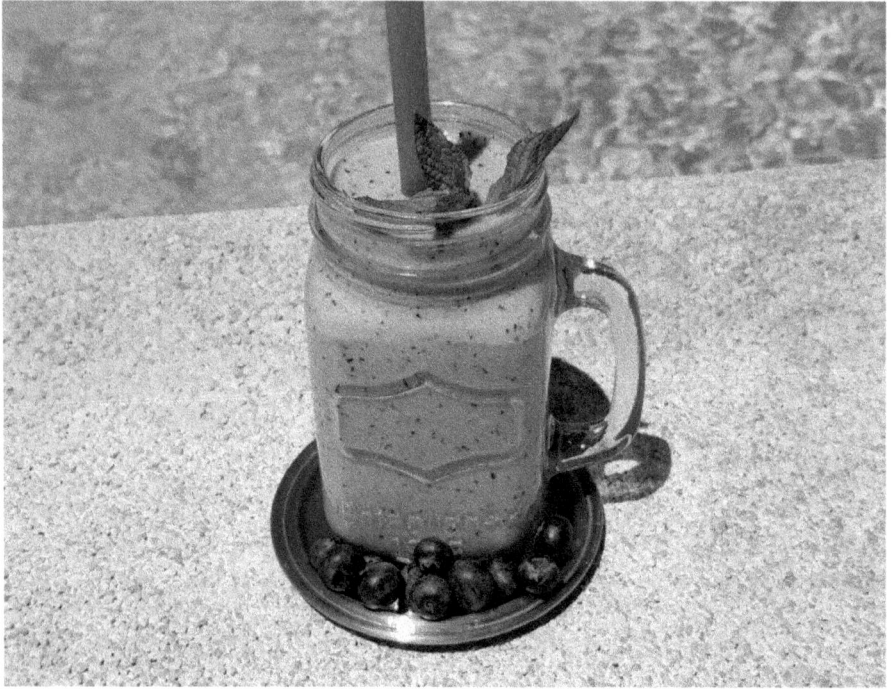

Herb-Topped Focaccia Preparation

Preparation Time: 20 minutes
Cooking Time: 2 hours
Servings: 10

Ingredients:

1 tbsp. dried rosemary or 3 tbsp. minced fresh
1 tbsp rosemary.
3 tbsp dried thyme minced fresh thyme leaves
½ cup extra-virgin olive oil
1 tsp. sugar
1 cup warm water
1 (¼-oz.) packet active dry yeast
2½ cups flour, divided
1 tsp salt

Directions:

1.In a small bowl, combine the rosemary and thyme with the olive oil.

2.In a large bowl, whisk together the sugar, water, and yeast. Let stand for 5 minutes.

3.Add 1 cup of flour, half of the olive oil mixture, and the salt to the large bowl mixture. Stir to combine.

4.Add the remaining 1½ cups flour to the large bowl. Using your hands, combine dough until it starts to pull away from the sides of the bowl.

5.Put the dough on a floured board or countertop and knead 10 to 12 times. Place the dough in a well-oiled bowl and cover with plastic wrap. Put it in a warm, dry space for 1 hour.

6.Oil a 9-by-13-inch baking pan. Turn the dough onto the baking pan, and using your hands gently push the dough out to fit the pan.

7.Using your fingers, make dimples into the dough. Evenly pour the remaining half of the olive oil mixture over the dough. Let the dough rise for another 30 minutes.

8.Preheat the oven to 450°F. Place the dough into the oven and let cook for 18 to 20 minutes, until you see it turn a golden brown.

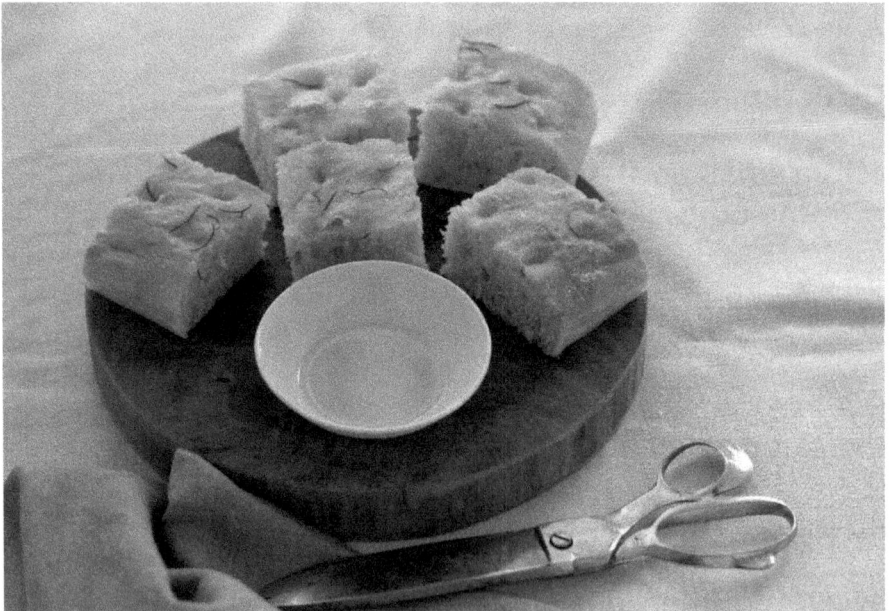

Caramelized Onion Flatbread with Arugula

Preparation Time: 10 minutes

Cooking Time: 25 minutes

Servings: 4

Ingredients:

4 tbsp. extra-virgin olive oil, divided
2 large onions, sliced into ¼-inch-thick slices
1 tsp. salt, divided
1 sheet puff pastry
1 (5-oz.) package goat cheese
8 oz. arugula
½ tsp. freshly ground black pepper

Directions:

1.Preheat the oven to 400°F.

2.In a large skillet over medium heat, cook 3 tbsp. olive oil, the onions, and ½ tsp. of salt, stirring, for 10 to 12 minutes, until the onions are translucent and golden brown.

3.To assemble, line a baking sheet with parchment paper. Lay the puff pastry flat on the parchment paper. Prick the middle of the puff pastry all over with a fork, leaving a ½-inch border.

4.Evenly distribute the onions on the pastry, leaving the border.

5.Crumble the goat cheese over the onions. Put the pastry in the oven to bake for 10 to 12 minutes, or until you see the border become golden brown.

6.Remove the pastry from the oven, set aside. In a medium bowl, add the arugula, remaining 1 tbsp. of olive oil, remaining ½ tsp. of salt, and ½ tsp. black pepper; toss to evenly dress the arugula.

7.Cut the pastry into even squares. Top the pastry with dressed arugula and serve.

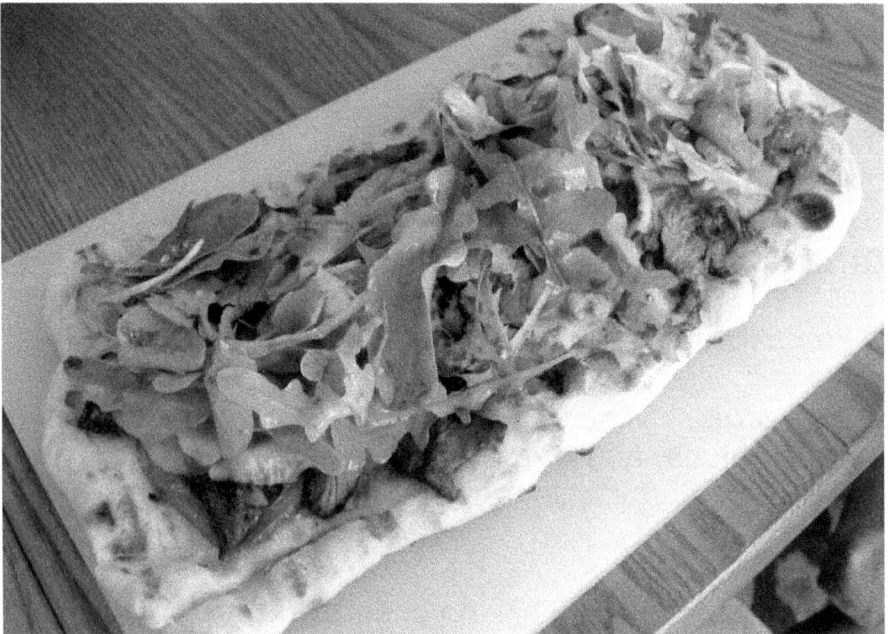

Balsamic Asparagus

Preparation Time: 10 minutes
Cooking Time: 15 minutes
Servings: 4

Ingredients:

3 tablespoons olive oil
3 garlic cloves, minced
2 tablespoons shallot, chopped
Salt and black pepper to the taste
2 teaspoons balsamic vinegar
1 and ½ pound asparagus, trimmed

Directions:

1.Heat a pan with the oil over medium-high heat, add the garlic and the shallot and sauté for 3 minutes.

2.Add the rest of the ingredients, cook for 12 minutes more, divide between plates and serve as a side dish.

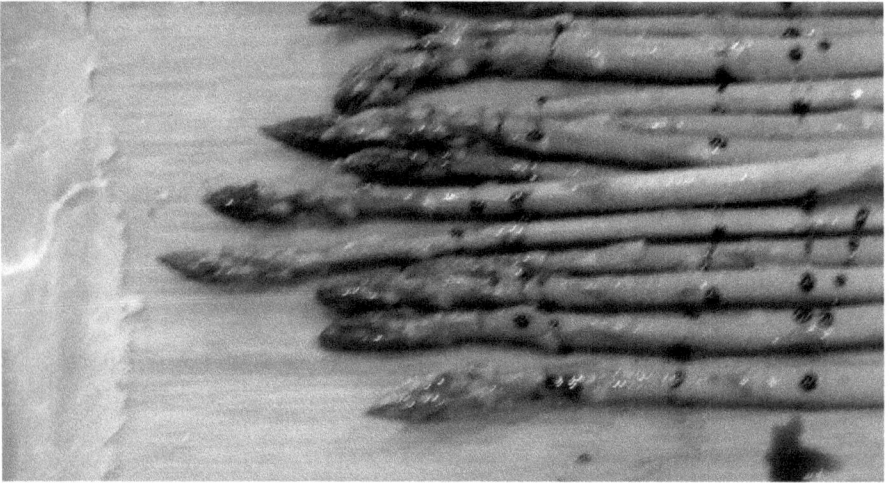

Lime Cucumber Mix

Preparation Time: 10 minutes
Cooking Time: 0 minutes
Servings: 8

Ingredients:

4 cucumbers, chopped
½ cup green bell pepper, chopped
1 yellow onion, chopped
1 chili pepper, chopped
1 garlic clove, minced
1 teaspoon parsley, chopped
2 tablespoons lime juice
1 tablespoon dill, chopped
Salt and black pepper to the taste
1 tablespoon olive oil

Directions:

1.In a large bowl, mix the cucumber with the bell peppers and the rest of the ingredients, toss and serve as a side dish.

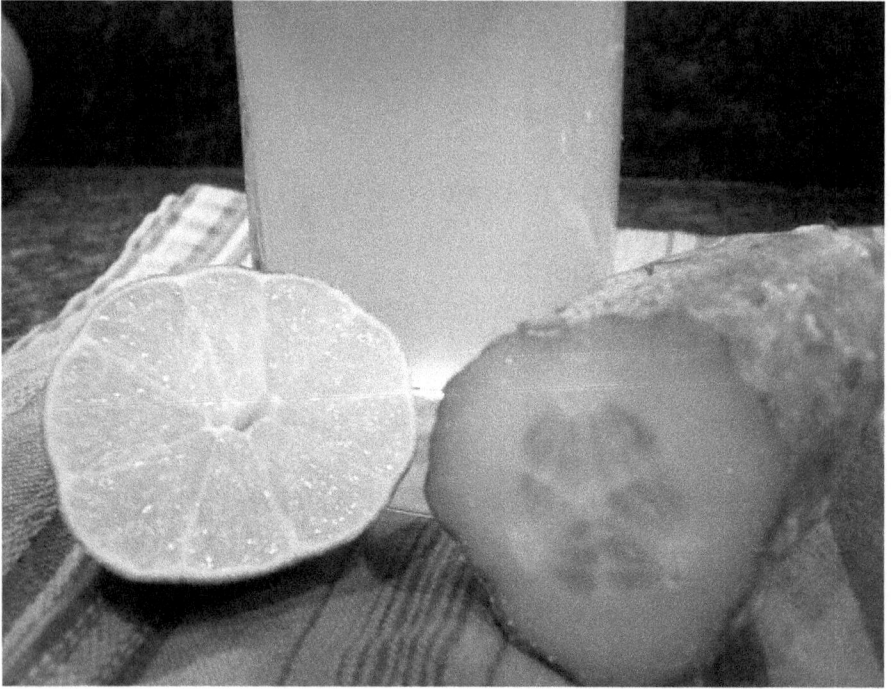

Walnuts Cucumber Mix

Preparation Time: 5 minutes
Cooking Time: 0 minutes
Servings: 2

Ingredients:

2 cucumbers, chopped
1 tablespoon olive oil
Salt and black pepper to the taste
1 red chili pepper, dried
1 tablespoon lemon juice
3 tablespoons walnuts, chopped
1 tablespoon balsamic vinegar
1 teaspoon chives, chopped

Directions:

1.In a bowl, mix the cucumbers with the oil and the rest of the ingredients, toss and serve as a side dish.

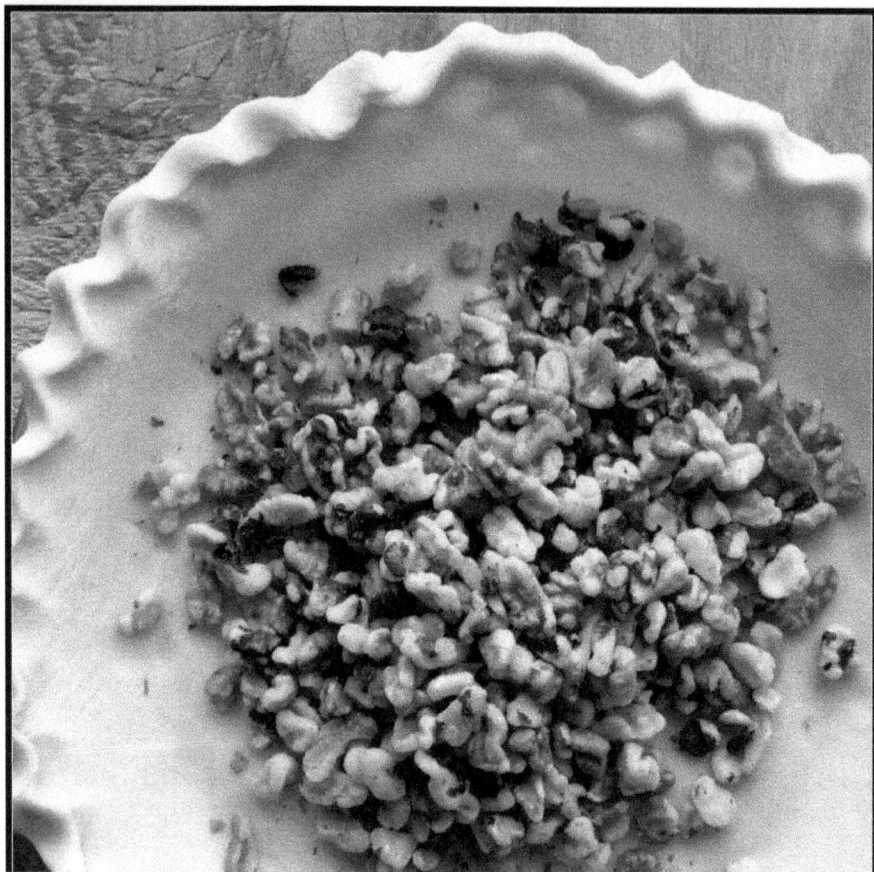

Cheesy Beet Salad

Preparation Time: 10 minutes
Cooking Time: 1 hour
Servings: 4

Ingredients:

4 beets, peeled and cut into wedges
3 tablespoons olive oil
Salt and black pepper to the taste
¼ cup lime juice
8 slices goat cheese, crumbled
1/3 cup walnuts, chopped
1 tablespoons chives, chopped

Directions:

1.In a roasting pan, combine the beets with the oil, salt and pepper, toss and bake at 400 degrees F for 1 hour.

2.Cool the beets down, transfer them to a bowl, add the rest of the ingredients, toss and serve as a side salad.

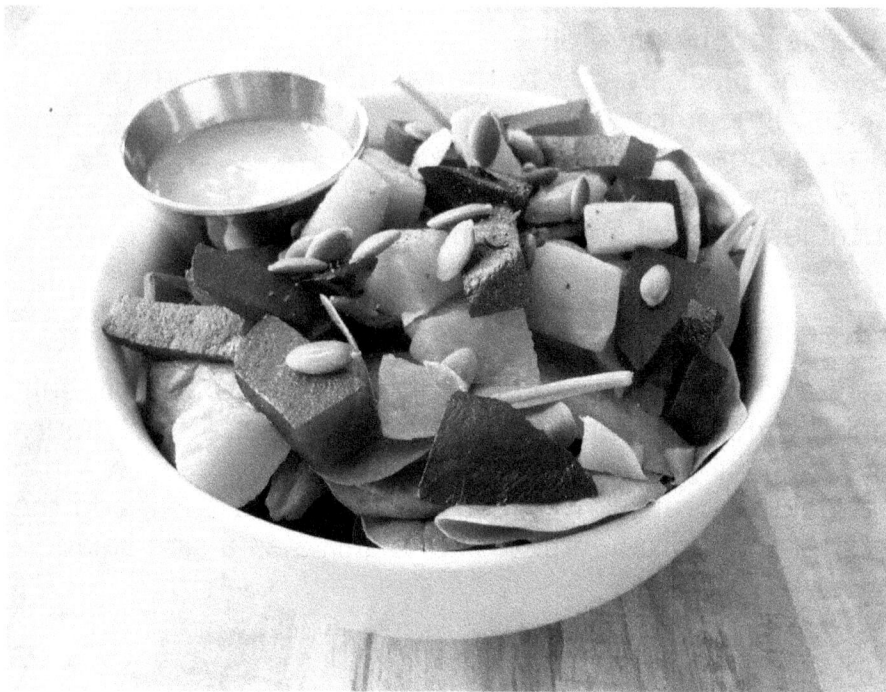

Rosemary Beets

Preparation Time: 10 minutes
Cooking Time: 20 minutes
Servings: 4

Ingredients:

4 medium beets, peeled and cubed
1/3 cup balsamic vinegar
1 teaspoon rosemary, chopped
1 garlic clove, minced
½ teaspoon Italian seasoning
1 tablespoon olive oil

Directions:

1.Heat a pan with the oil over medium heat, add the beets and the rest of the ingredients, toss, and cook for 20 minutes.

2.Divide the mix between plates and serve as a side dish.

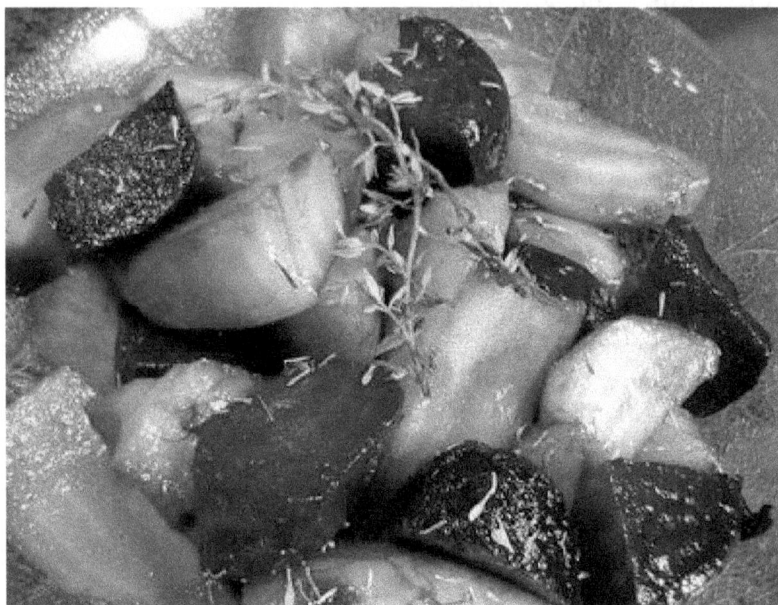

Squash and Tomatoes Mix

Preparation Time: 10 minutes
Cooking Time: 20 minutes
Servings: 6

Ingredients:

5 medium squash, cubed
A pinch of salt and black pepper
3 tablespoons olive oil
1 cup pine nuts, toasted
¼ cup goat cheese, crumbled
6 tomatoes, cubed
½ yellow onion, chopped
2 tablespoons cilantro, chopped
2 tablespoons lemon juice

Directions:

1.Heat a pan with the oil over medium heat, add the onion and pine nuts and cook for 3 minutes.

2.Add the squash and the rest of the ingredients, cook everything for 15 minutes, divide between plates and serve as a side dish.

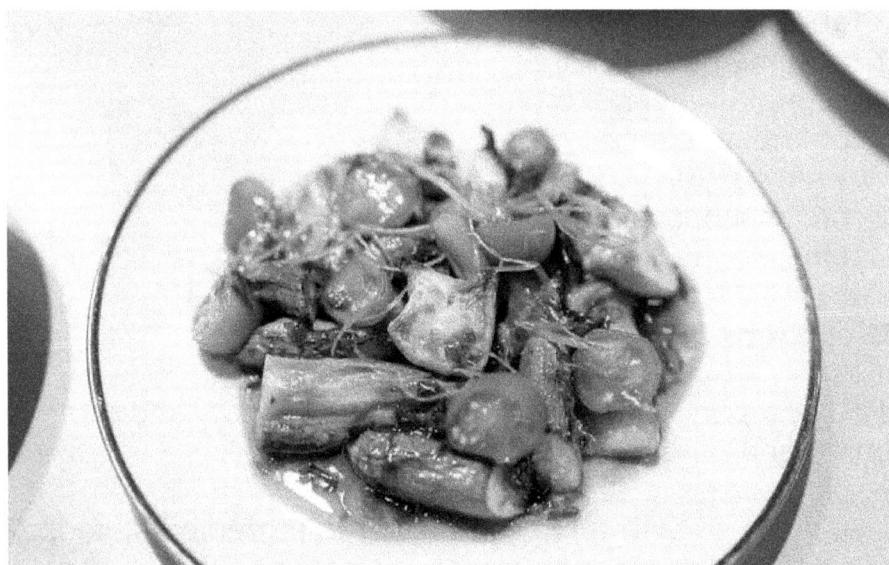

Balsamic Eggplant Mix

Preparation Time: 10 minutes
Cooking Time: 20 minutes
Servings: 6

Ingredients:

1/3 cup chicken stock
2 tablespoons balsamic vinegar
A pinch of salt and black pepper
1 tablespoon lime juice
2 big eggplants, sliced
1 tablespoon rosemary, chopped
¼ cup cilantro, chopped
2 tablespoons olive oil

Directions:

1.In a roasting pan, combine the eggplants with the stock, the vinegar and the rest of the ingredients, introduce the pan in the oven and bake at 390 degrees F for 20 minutes.

2.Divide the mix between plates and serve as a side dish.

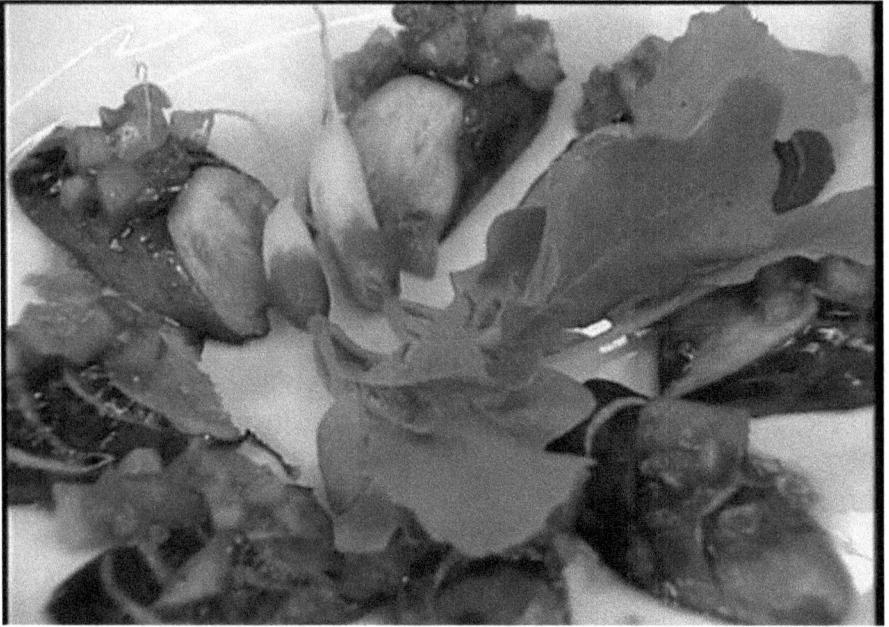

Sage Barley Mix

Preparation Time: 10 minutes
Cooking Time: 45 minutes
Servings: 4

Ingredients:

1 tablespoon olive oil
1 red onion, chopped
1 tablespoon leaves, chopped
1 garlic clove, minced
14 ounces barley
½ tablespoon parmesan, grated
6 cups veggie stock
Salt and black pepper to the taste

Directions:

1.Heat a pan with the oil over medium heat, add the onion and garlic, stir and sauté for 5 minutes.

2.Add the sage, barley and the rest of the ingredients except the parmesan, stir, bring to a simmer and cook for 40 minutes,

3.Add the parmesan, stir, and divide between plates.

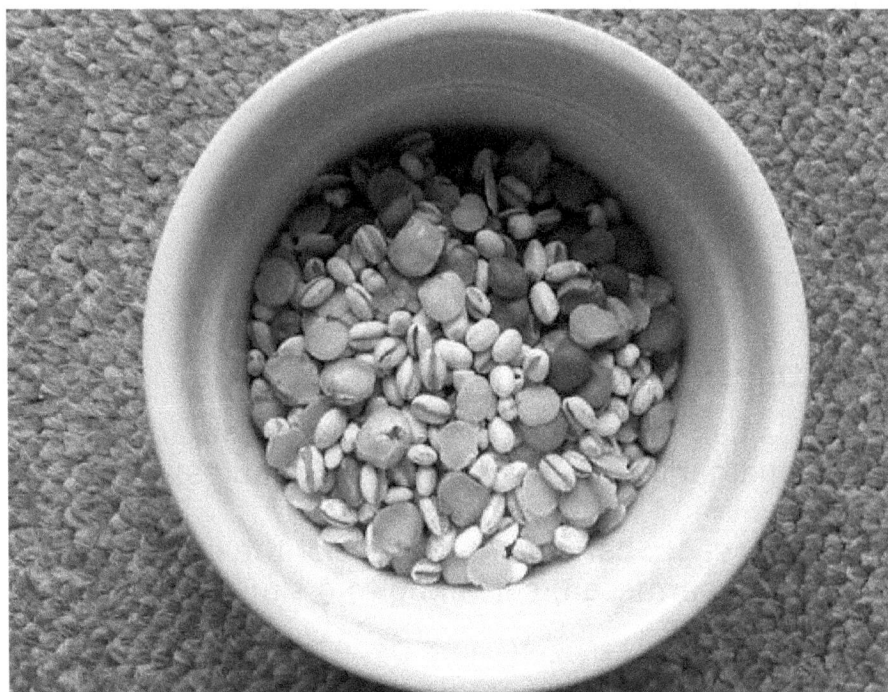

Cucumber Bites

Preparation Time: 10 minutes
Cooking Time: 0 minutes
Servings: 12

Ingredients:

1English cucumber, sliced into
32pounds 10 oz. hummus
16herry tomatoes, halved
1tbsp. parsley, chopped
1 oz. feta cheese, crumbled

Directioms:

1.Spread the hummus on each cucumber round, divide the tomato halves on each, sprinkle the cheese and parsley on to and serve as an appetizer.

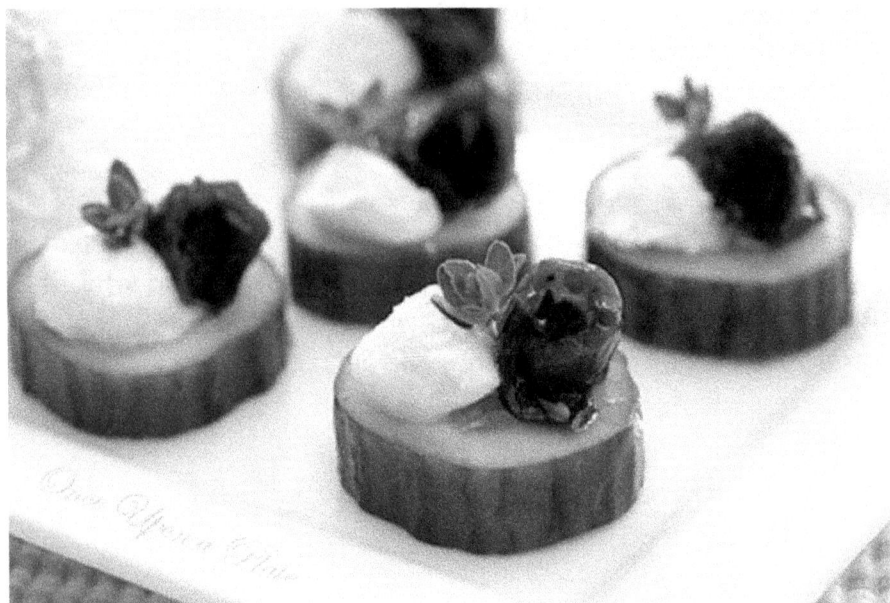

Stuffed Avocado Preparation

Time: 10 minutes
Cooking Time: 0 minute
Servings: 2

Ingredients:

1 avocado, halved and pitted
10 oz. canned tuna, drained
2 tbsp. sun-dried tomatoes, chopped 1 and ½ tbsp.
basil pesto
2tbsp. black olives, pitted and chopped
Salt and black pepper to the taste
2tsp. pine nuts, toasted and chopped
1 tbsp. basil, chopped

Directions:

1.In a bowl, combine the tuna with the sun-dried
tomatoes and the rest of the ingredients except the
avocado and stir.

2.Stuff the avocado halves with the tuna mix and serve
as an appetizer.

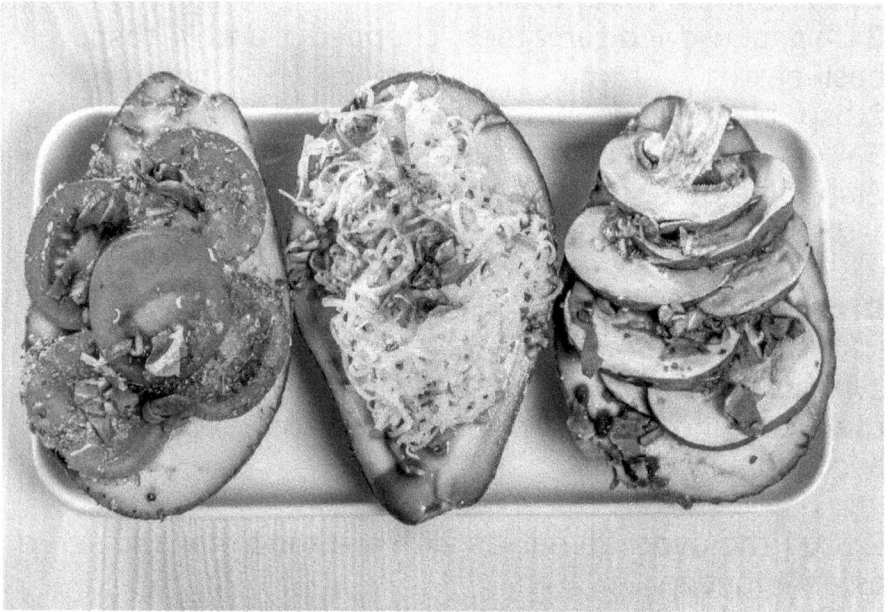

www.ingramcontent.com/pod-product-compliance
Lightning Source LLC
Chambersburg PA
CBHW050749030426
42336CB00012B/1726